Introduction

Not only in relation to illness, but also in the day-to-day news from many sources we face medical terms only partly understood or not understood at all. With over 2,000 carefully chosen entries this dictionary aims to be practical and up to date for the home and for medical ancillary workers. Where necessary a more extended explanation supplements the definition itself. Line illustrations are included wherever they can help to make the terms clearer.

A very full system of cross references assists the reader to find his way from one related topic to another. It also allows the greatest amount of information to be given in a small space. Thus many of the entries contain words which are themselves defined elsewhere. These are set in small capital letters so that they can be easily found in their proper alphabetical place.

Terms which are made up of two words, for example, *acute abdomen* or *mucous membrane*, are not entered under their key words (*abdomen* or *membrane*), but alphabetically under their full titles. Many entries carry a cross reference to more general ones which have illustrations. For example, *cornea* refers to *eye* and *femur* to *skeleton*: the labelled diagrams under *eye* and *skeleton* are much more informative than mere words could be.

Used in this way the dictionary will cover almost all the medical terms likely to interest or puzzle the layman and perhaps also clear up quite a few misconceptions.

A.S.P.

a- A prefix meaning 'absent', 'not' or 'without'.

A

abdomen The large space between the ribs and diaphragm above and the pelvis below. The back and sides have the bony protection of the vertebral column, ribs and pelvic bones, but the front has only the softness of muscles and skin. The main contents are the liver, stomach, intestines, kidneys, spleen, pancreas and bladder and, in women, the uterus and ovaries.

abducens nerve The sixth CRANIAL NERVE, it supplies the muscles which move the eyeball.

abduction Movement which draws a limb or part of the body away from the mid-line of the body. (Compare ADDUCTION)

abortifacient An instrument or drug causing an abortion.

abortion The ending of a pregnancy and the expulsion of the foetus before it is likely to survive birth, assessed as 28 weeks after the beginning of the last period.
Threatened abortion: Onset of bleeding in early pregnancy, with possibility that treatment will maintain pregnancy.
Inevitable abortion: Sustained bleeding and medical signs indicating that treatment would be ineffective.

abrasion A graze or superficial wound to the skin caused by rubbing or scraping.

abreaction A process in psychiatry of reducing tension in a patient by making him aware of feelings or incidents which have been causing him stress by lying suppressed in his unconscious mind.

abscess A localized collection of PUS in any part of the body.

abulia In psychiatry absence of will power.

a.c. A prescription indication meaning 'before food' – the initials of the Latin words 'ante cibum'.

A.C. An abbreviation for air conduction. (see RINNE TEST)

accessory nerve The eleventh CRANIAL NERVE, it supplies the muscles of the neck and shoulders.

accommodation The ability of the eye to adjust its lens to focus on objects at various distances.

acetabulum The cup-shaped part of the PELVIS into which the rounded head of the FEMUR fits, to form the hip joint.

acetone A chemical with a characteristic odour resembling that of nail varnish. In the body it is produced only in some abnormal conditions, such as severe DIABETES, and can then be detected in the urine (acetonuria).

acetyl salicylic acid The chemical name for ASPIRIN.

achalasia The failure to relax of the muscle surrounding the opening of the OESOPHAGUS into the stomach, thus preventing food from entering the stomach.

Achilles tendon The large tendon at the back of the lower leg attaching the calf muscles to the heel.

achlorhydria Absence of hydrochloric acid normally present in the stomach. The acid plays a part in digestion and in the absorption of iron from foods. (Compare HYPOCHLORHYDRIA)

achondroplasia A condition, present at birth, in which there is defective growth of the long bones of the limbs. This results in dwarfism, in which the individual has a normal trunk and head but very short arms and legs.

The Hamlyn Pocket
Medical
Dictionary

The Hamlyn Pocket

Medical Dictionary

Dr A S Playfair

Hamlyn

London · New York · Sydney · Toronto

First published in 1980 by
The Hamlyn Publishing Group Limited
London · New York · Sydney · Toronto
Astronaut House, Feltham, Middlesex, England

ISBN 0 600 36311 2

Printed in Great Britain by
Hazell Watson & Viney Ltd, Aylesbury, Bucks

acidosis A reduction in the normal degree of alkalinity of the blood and body fluids, altering the acid–alkali balance in the body. This can arise in various ways, for example as a result of kidney failure, respiration difficulties, diabetes, starvation, heavy diarrhoea and some forms of poisoning.

acne Overactivity of the SEBACEOUS GLANDS of the skin producing excess sebum which blocks the gland opening with a small black plug – the blackhead or comedone. Blackheads tend to form infected pimples and are very common on the face and back of adolescents.

acoustic Relating to hearing or to sound.

acoustic neuroma A benign tumour of the sheath of the auditory nerve. (See CRANIAL NERVES)

acquired A term generally used to describe a permanent impairment of health which is neither CONGENITAL nor HEREDITARY.

acromegaly A slowly developing condition in which there is excessive secretion of the growth HORMONE by the PITUITARY GLAND. This produces enlargement and thickening of the hands, feet and head.

acromion The tip of the scapula (see SKELETON) which forms the point of the shoulder.

acroparaesthesia A disease characterized by sudden attacks of pain in the arm and tingling or numbness of the fingers.

acrophobia Fear of heights.

A.C.T.H. An abbreviation for ADRENOCORTICOTROPIC HORMONE.

actinomycosis An infection caused by a species of
FUNGUS. It generally affects the mouth, lungs and
intestines, where it forms abscesses.

active exercise and movements Those in which the
motions are performed under a person's voluntary
control. (Compare PASSIVE EXERCISE AND MOVEMENTS)

acupuncture A treatment of Chinese origin which consists
of inserting needles into the skin and gently rotating
them. Insertions are made at points of the body which
are considered to be specific for the disease, but not
necessarily in its area. Acupuncture is also used to
produce anaesthesia.

acute A term used to describe an illness of sudden onset
and short duration and sometimes of considerable
severity. The opposite is CHRONIC.

acute abdomen A term used by doctors for any sudden
severe condition within the ABDOMEN needing urgent
LAPAROTOMY. It often implies that the exact diagnosis is
uncertain until the operation allows inspection of the
abdominal contents.

addiction A craving for a potentially harmful drug with
increased bodily tolerance for it in large doses and the
likelihood of unpleasant effects if it is suddenly
withdrawn.

Addison's disease A disease due to inadequate secretion of
certain HORMONES by the ADRENAL GLANDS. Among its
features are weakness, ANAEMIA, low blood pressure,
nausea and patchy dark discoloration of the skin.

adduction Movement which brings a limb or part of the
body closer to the mid-line of the body. (Compare
ABDUCTION)

aden(o)- A prefix meaning 'relating to a gland'.

adenitis Inflammation of a gland.

adenocarcinoma CARCINOMA of GLAND tissue.

adenoid A mass of lymphatic tissue high on the back of the PHARYNX. It provides protection against infection spreading from the mouth and nose.

adenoma A tumour, generally BENIGN, of GLAND tissue.

adenovirus A VIRUS often associated with sore throats and common colds.

adhesion An abnormal joining together of membranes or organs. This may follow inflammation or wound healing, with adhering tissue forming in the areas involved.

adipose tissue The layer of CONNECTIVE TISSUE under the skin which contains and stores fat.

adiposis dolorosa or **Dercum's disease** An illness of women characterized by scattered painful nodules of fatty deposits.

adiposo-genital syndrome see **Fröhlich's syndrome**

adnexa The accessory structures of an organ, for example the FALLOPIAN TUBES, ligaments and OVARIES in the region of the UTERUS.

adrenal glands or **suprarenal glands** Situated at the upper end of each kidney, the two adrenal glands produce important HORMONES like ADRENALINE and CORTICOSTEROIDS.

adrenaline A HORMONE secreted by the ADRENAL GLAND. By stimulating the SYMPATHETIC NERVOUS SYSTEM it

11

increases heart action, blood pressure and rate of
breathing and relaxes bowel activity and the muscles
round the air tubes.

adrenocorticotrophic hormone A HORMONE secreted by
the PITUITARY GLAND which stimulates the ADRENAL GLAND
to produce CORTICOSTEROIDS.

aerobe A MICRO-ORGANISM which requires the presence of
oxygen to live.

aerophagia The swallowing of air, often a habitual TIC.

aetiology The cause of a disease.

afebrile Without a fever; of normal temperature.

affect The feeling experienced with an emotion, for
example, pleasure or distress.

afterbirth see **placenta**

after-pains Painful awareness of the normal rhythmic
contractions of the UTERUS which follow childbirth.

agglutination The clumping of BACTERIA, thus rendering
them inactive, caused by the introduction of ANTIBODIES.
The term is also used to describe the effect on red blood
cells when different BLOOD GROUPS are mixed.

agnosia Failure to recognize familiar sights, sounds, or
other sensations, due generally to a lesion of the brain.

agoraphobia An abnormal fear of being out alone and in
open spaces.

agranulocytosis A deficiency in the number of certain
white blood cells. (See LEUCOCYTES)

A.I.D. see **artificial insemination**

A.I.H. see **artificial insemination**

air conduction see **Rinne test**

albinism The condition of a person (an albino) born with a lack of normal body pigment. The albino has very pink skin, white hair and pink eyes.

albumin One of the various complex PROTEINS that form the main chemical composition of all living organisms.

albuminuria The presence of ALBUMIN in the urine. This is an abnormal condition and may indicate a disorder of the kidney.

alcoholism Addiction to and dependence on alcoholic drinks.

aldosterone A corticosteroid HORMONE secreted by the ADRENAL GLAND. It regulates the balance of sodium and potassium in the body.

alexia Word blindness or inability to understand written or printed words, a condition caused by a disorder of the brain.

alimentary canal The whole DIGESTIVE TRACT extending from the mouth to the anus.

alkaloids A large group of compounds with potent effects found in plants. Some are used in medicine, such as caffeine, morphine and codeine. Other alkaloid drugs have been made synthetically.

alkalosis An abnormal increase in the alkalinity of the blood and body fluids. One of its effects is severe cramp in the muscles.

alkaptonuria A CONGENITAL condition in which dark pigment colours the urine and is deposited in the body.

allergen

allergen A substance which can produce an ALLERGY.

allergy Abnormal sensitivity to foreign substances. The introduction into the body of potentially harmful substances, ANTIGENS, stimulates production of defence material, ANTIBODIES, to neutralize them. In allergic conditions antibodies may be formed against ordinary substances, such as foods, pollen or feathers, or against drugs. (See also HISTAMINE)

allo– A prefix meaning 'other' or 'different'.

allograft see **grafting**

allopathy A system of treatment with drugs which in a healthy person produce symptoms opposite to those of the disease. (Compare HOMEOPATHY)

alopecia Loss of hair; baldness.

alveolus (plural, *alveoli)* A small cavity or socket, in particular one of the many minute air sacs of the lungs where an exchange of gases takes place, oxygen being carried into the blood and carbon dioxide removed. (See LUNGS)

amaurosis Blindness in the absence of any obvious abnormality of the eye.

amaurotic familial idiocy A hereditary disease marked by brain damage, mental defects, paralysis and blindness.

ambivalence Co-existence in the mind of contradictory opinions or feelings about a person or object.

amblyopia Dimness of vision without any detectable lesion of the eye itself, for example, as the result of a brain lesion, and therefore not correctable by the use of glasses.

ambulatory Of a patient, able to walk.

amenorrhoea Absence of menstrual periods. It may be called 'primary' when periods never appear or 'secondary' when they cease after having previously been present.

amentia Mental subnormality.

amino-acids Chemicals which unite together to form the more complex PROTEINS. The body can synthesize some of them for its needs, but others must come from food.

amnesia Loss of memory.

amniocentesis The use of a syringe and needle to take a sample of the AMNIOTIC FLUID during pregnancy in order to test certain health factors in the unborn baby.

amnion The membranous bag in the UTERUS containing the AMNIOTIC FLUID.

amniotic fluid The fluid in which the FOETUS floats in the womb.

amoeba (plural, *amoebae*) A single-celled animal.

amoebiasis Infection with a type of amoeba parasitic in man.

amoebic dysentery Dysentery caused by infection with parasitic amoebae.

amputation Surgical or accidental removal of a limb or part of a limb.

anabolism The process by which more complex chemical substances are built up in the body from simpler ones. (Compare CATABOLISM)

anaemia Reduction in the number of the red blood cells (ERYTHROCYTES) in the circulation or in the HAEMOGLOBIN they contain, and consequently of the oxygen-carrying capacity of the blood.

anaerobe A MICRO-ORGANISM which lives without oxygen, that is, in the absence of air.

anaerobic Relating to the absence of oxygen.

anaesthesia The absence of bodily sensation. A general anaesthetic is administered to give total loss of consciousness. A local anaesthetic can be injected or applied as a liquid or ointment in order to numb a selected part.

analeptic A drug which acts as a restorative or a stimulant.

analgesia Absence of sensitivity to pain. Analgesic drugs are given to reduce pain.

anaphylaxis An extremely severe reaction to a foreign protein or other substance to which the body has already become sensitized. (See ALLERGY)

anastomosis An abnormal connection or, as treatment, a surgically created connection between two hollow structures, such as between blood vessels or parts of the digestive tract.

Ancylostoma see **hookworm**

androgen A substance which increases the male characteristics of the body, for example TESTOSTERONE.

anencephaly Congenital absence of or minimal development of the brain, a defect incompatible with life.

aneurysm The swelling or bulging of a blood vessel, together with the weakening of its wall. A rare special case is the *dissecting aneurysm* where a tear in the inner lining of an artery is followed by the diffusion of blood between the layers of the walls, a condition causing intense pain.

angina or **angina pectoris** A pain in the front of the chest, behind the breastbone, often spreading to the neck and shoulders. It arises from inadequate oxygen supply to the heart. It is particularly liable to occur during physical effort by a person in whom the arteries to the heart wall muscles are narrow and inelastic; the blood supply cannot keep pace with the need of the heart in exertion. The condition is quite unrelated to VINCENT'S ANGINA.

angio– A prefix meaning 'vessel' and usually referring to blood vessels.

angioedema Another term for ANGIONEUROTIC OEDEMA.

angiography The examination of blood vessels by injecting them with a liquid which is opaque to X-rays. The resulting picture is an angiogram.

angioma A tumour or swelling made up of a collection of blood vessels. On the skin it can form a NAEVUS.

angioneurotic oedema Recurrent attacks of OEDEMA of some parts of the skin or of the MUCOUS MEMBRANE.

anhidrotic A preparation used to reduce perspiration.

ankle jerk The REFLEX downward jerk of the foot when the tendon at the back of the ankle is tapped sharply.

ankylosis Immobility of a joint due to abnormal fusion of its bones.

ankylostomiasis A disease caused by HOOKWORMS in the intestines and characterized by anaemia and malnutrition.

anorexia Loss of appetite.

anorexia nervosa An emotional condition associated with fear of being or becoming overweight, leading to prolonged loss of appetite and emaciation. It affects mainly young women.

anosmia Absence of the sense of smell.

anoxia Absence or shortage of oxygen in the body.

antacid Any medicine used to reduce excess acid in the stomach.

antecubital Relating to the area in the fold of the elbow.

antepartum Before labour and childbirth.

anthracosis Discoloration of the lungs caused by deposits of soot and coal dust. The condition can be found in coal miners and city dwellers and is generally harmless.

anthrax An infection caused by a BACILLUS, and generally caught from animals or through contact with hides. It can produce severe pus-filled eruptions of the skin or it can give PNEUMONIA or GASTROENTERITIS.

antibiotic A chemical substance, such as penicillin, derived from a MICRO-ORGANISM, usually a FUNGUS, and used as a drug to prevent the growth of or to kill harmful micro-organisms.

antibodies Defensive substances produced in the body specifically to neutralize or render inactive foreign

substances (ANTIGENS), including bacteria. (See also
ALLERGY)

anticoagulant An agent which delays, reduces or prevents
the COAGULATION of blood.

antidepressant A drug used to relieve mental depression.

antigen A substance foreign to the body which, when
introduced into it, stimulates the production of
ANTIBODIES. (See also ALLERGY)

antihistamine A preparation designed to counteract the
effect of HISTAMINE in the body. (See ALLERGY)

antipyretic A preparation which reduces a fever.

antiseptic A preparation used to destroy or arrest the
growth of harmful MICRO-ORGANISMS.

antiserum SERUM from an animal which has developed
ANTIBODIES against a bacterial infection. It can be used to
protect man against that infection or in laboratory tests
on bacteria.

antitoxin An ANTIBODY produced in the body as reaction
to the toxin or poison of an infecting MICRO-ORGANISM or
to the bites of animals like snakes. Injections of SERUM
containing antitoxin can be used as treatment of some
infections.

antitussive A medicine used to reduce coughing.

antivenin SERUM containing antitoxins against poison
from the bites or stings of animals like snakes or
scorpions.

antrum A cavity in an organ of the body, in particular one
of the air SINUSES in the nose, which is also called the
maxillary sinus.

anuria Absence of urine formation by the kidneys or, through blockage of the URINARY TRACT, failure to pass urine.

anus The opening of the last part of the DIGESTIVE TRACT, the RECTUM, to the outside.

anxiety In psychiatry a NEUROSIS with emotional disturbance characterized by fears ranging from unease to dread, unrelated to or out of proportion to any real cause. (See also PHOBIA)

aorta The largest ARTERY of the body, beginning at the heart and descending into the abdomen. From its branches the whole body receives its blood supply. (See CIRCULATION OF THE BLOOD)

aperient A purgative.

aphasia Loss of the power of understanding or expressing oneself by written and spoken words, gestures or symbols. This is generally due to damage to the brain centres concerned, and is not related to intelligence.

aphonia Loss of power to produce vocal sounds.

aphrodisiac Any substance which stimulates sexual desire or increases potency.

aphtha (plural, *aphthae*) A small ulcer in the mouth.

aplastic anaemia ANAEMIA due to the body's gross underproduction of RED BLOOD CELLS.

apnoea Absence of or cessation of breathing.

apoplexy see **stroke**

appendix A thin tube-like appendage of the CAECUM about three inches long. It has no known function. Inflammation of the appendix (appendicitis) is usually treated by surgical removal (appendicectomy).

apraxia Inability to perform purposeful movements in a patient not suffering from paralysis or loss of sensation.

aqueous humour A fluid in the front of the eyeball filling the space between the lens and the cornea. (See EYE)

arachnoid The middle one of the three MENINGES which cover the brain and spinal cord.

arcus senilis A thin dark ring on the CORNEA of the eye around the IRIS. Found in elderly people, it is harmless.

areola The coloured, circular area of skin around the nipple of the breast.

areolar tissue One type of CONNECTIVE TISSUE.

Argyll Robertson pupil A condition of the eye in which the PUPIL reacts to light but does not, as is normal, change size with ACCOMMODATION.

arrhythmia A variation in the normal rhythm of the heart beat. Some arrhythmias are of no significance as far as the health of the heart is concerned.

artefact A feature made by man; something artificial which does not occur naturally.

arteriography ANGIOGRAPHY of an artery.

arteriole The smallest size of ARTERY.

arteriosclerosis Thickening of the wall and narrowing of the channel of the arteries, accompanied by loss of elasticity. This can lead to high blood pressure and extra work for the heart.

artery Any blood vessel carrying blood from the direction of the heart towards the other parts of the body. (See CIRCULATION OF THE BLOOD)

arthritis Inflammation of a JOINT.

arthrodesis An operation to fuse a JOINT in its most useful position. Though this stops movement it relieves the intense pain caused by severe inflammation and restores some efficiency to the joint.

arthropathy Any disease of a JOINT.

arthroplasty An operation to reconstruct and improve a damaged or diseased JOINT or to replace it with an artificial one.

arthroscopy The examination of the inside of a JOINT by means of a special optical tube.

articulation A JOINT or juncture of bones.

artificial insemination Artificial introduction of viable SPERMATOZOA into the VAGINA of a woman who wants a child but whose attempts to conceive have failed, either because of her husband's inability to ejaculate in her vagina or because his semen is inadequate. A.I.H. (artificial insemination from the husband's semen) may be successful.

    If the husband's semen is not suitable then A.I.D. (artificial insemination from the semen of a donor) can be considered in special circumstances. The donor will be unknown to the couple.

artificial kidney see **kidney machine**

asbestosis PNEUMOCONIOSIS caused by inhalation of asbestos dust. One risk from asbestosis is lung cancer.

ascariasis INFESTATION of the intestines with a type of roundworm, the ascaris.

ascites Abnormal accumulation of fluid in the abdominal cavity; a form of DROPSY.

ascorbic acid see **vitamins**

asepsis Freedom from infection and the presence of MICRO-ORGANISMS.

aspergillosis Infection with a harmful species of aspergillus, a type of fungus.

asphyxia Suffocation or choking.

asphyxia neonatorum In a newborn baby, failure to breathe or difficulty in breathing.

aspiration Withdrawal of fluid, for example, from a cavity in the body by suction, as with a syringe or through a tube.

aspirin A white crystalline substance used as an analgesic to relieve the pain caused by headache, rheumatism, etc.

astereognosis Inability to identify objects by feeling them.

asthenia Weakness; loss of energy.

asthma A condition characterized by recurring attacks of difficult breathing and of breathlessness due to contraction of the air tubes and the production of sticky mucus within them. An ALLERGY is the major cause but INFECTION and emotion may also be important factors. This is bronchial asthma and unrelated to CARDIAC ASTHMA.

astigmatism Partial blurring of vision due to some irregularity in the CORNEA, through which the light passes at the front of the eyeball. (See EYE)

astringent A preparation causing shrinkage of a body surface (skin or MUCOUS MEMBRANE) to which it is applied. It acts by contracting the blood vessels.

ataractic see **tranquillizer**

ataxia Failure of the normal coordination between the actions of muscles, making walking movements, for example, difficult and jerky. The cause lies in a defect in those parts of the nervous system which govern REFLEXES and give unconscious signals concerning muscle position.

atelectasis 1 Incomplete intake of air and expansion of a baby's lung at birth. **2** A condition in which a lung or part of a lung becomes airless owing to an obstruction in the air tube leading to it.

atheroma A deposit of fatty material (chiefly CHOLESTEROL) within an artery on its lining wall. This narrows the artery and reduces the blood supply to the organ it serves. It also carries the risk of THROMBUS formation at the site. Faulty diet and smoking are considered to play some part in atheroma formation.

atherosclerosis A form of ARTERIOSCLEROSIS associated with ATHEROMA deposits.

athetosis Repetitive, purposeless and involuntary movements in the limbs, especially the arms and hands, resulting from brain disorder. It is seen in some forms of CEREBRAL PALSY.

athlete's foot An infectious disease of the skin of the foot caused by a FUNGUS.

atlas The first VERTEBRA of the spine, on which the skull rests. (See SKELETON)

atony Weakness, for example, of muscle; lack of normal strength.

atopy An ALLERGIC reaction, especially one that develops in a different place from the part where the sensitizing ALLERGEN came in contact with the body, such as the formation of a rash on the arms and trunk after the swallowing or inhaling of the allergen.

atresia Absence of or abnormal closure of a passage or orifice in the body, for example, the ANUS, VAGINA, OESOPHAGUS or a blood vessel. It is generally CONGENITAL.

atrial Relating to the heart; AURICULAR.

atrio-ventricular node see **heart**

atrium Another name for the AURICLE of the HEART.

atrophy Shrinkage; wasting away.

A.T.S. An abbreviation for anti-TETANUS SERUM.

attenuation A decrease in the virulence of live BACTERIA which permits them to retain their other characteristics for use in vaccines.

audiogram A chart showing the results of AUDIOMETRY on a patient.

audiometry A method of testing and measuring the hearing sensitivity of an ear to sound waves on different frequencies.

auditory nerve The eighth CRANIAL NERVE, it controls the sense of hearing and balance.

aura A warning sensation or premonition some patients experience before an attack of MIGRAINE or EPILEPSY.

aural Relating to the ear.

auricle 1 The outer, visible part of the ear. **2** The antechamber or collecting chamber on each side of the HEART, receiving on the left blood from the lungs and on the right that from the rest of the body.

auricular Relating to the AURICLE of the HEART.

auricular fibrillation FIBRILLATION of the AURICLES of the HEART. Since the pumping VENTRICLES of the heart are to a certain extent governed by the action of the auricles this produces completely irregular and weakened heart beats.

auscultation Listening to sounds made by organs in the body, such as the lungs, heart and intestines, as an aid to DIAGNOSIS. This is usually done with a STETHOSCOPE.

autism A condition marked by a self-centred withdrawal from one's surroundings. It appears in the very young child and persists to a greater or lesser extent as the child grows up. Development of speech, of gestures, of understanding and of personal relationships is often severely limited, and the child may repetitively perform meaningless actions. The cause is not fully understood.

autistic Suffering from AUTISM.

autograft see **grafting**

auto–immune diseases Several illnesses are believed to be related to the body's abnormal reaction to some of its own TISSUES, behaving as if they were ANTIGENS and producing ANTIBODIES against them (see ALLERGY). This damages the tissues and is called 'auto-immunity', though 'auto-allergy' would be a more accurate name.
    Possible auto-immune diseases include RHEUMATOID ARTHRITIS, some forms of NEPHRITIS, PERNICIOUS ANAEMIA, ULCERATIVE COLITIS and MYASTHENIA GRAVIS.

autonomic nervous system A system of nerves throughout the body functioning outside conscious control and regulating such features as heartbeat, blood pressure, the work of the intestines and the reaction of the eyes to light. Its two divisions are the *sympathetic*, which in general stimulates the body to activity and prepares it for emergencies, and the *parasympathetic*, which covers routine functions at rest, such as digestive processes. Many organs, like the heart, are under the balancing control of both systems.

autopsy Post-mortem examination, that is, dissection of the body of someone who has died from disease or injury in order to investigate in detail any abnormalities in the body and the factors contributing to death.

avascular Without a blood supply.

avascular necrosis The death of a tissue through disruption of its blood supply, for example, the death of an injured bone whose arteries have been severely damaged.

axilla The armpit.

axis The second VERTEBRA of the spine. (See SKELETON)

azoospermia Absence of SPERMATOZOA in the SEMEN.

Babinski test see **plantar response**

B

bacillus A rod-shaped BACTERIUM.

backbone The VERTEBRAL COLUMN.

bacteria A very large and varied group of single-celled MICRO-ORGANISMS which multiply by splitting into two.

bacteriaemia

They range from the useful, which help in the conditioning of soil, through the harmless to those producing disease.

In medicine their basic classification depends on shape as seen through the microscope. Cocci are spherical, bacilli are straight rods, vibrios are curved rods and spirilla or spirochaetes are spirals.

bacteriaemia The presence of BACTERIA in the blood.

bacterial endocarditis see **subacute bacterial endocarditis**

bactericide A preparation or process which kills BACTERIA.

bacteriology The scientific study of BACTERIA.

bacteriostasis A preparation or process that inhibits the growth or multiplication of BACTERIA.

bacterium The singular of BACTERIA.

bacteriuria The presence of BACTERIA in the urine.

Baghdad sore see **Leishmaniasis**

Baker's cyst A swelling at the back of the knee joint caused by a bulge of the SYNOVIAL MEMBRANE.

B.A.L. An abbreviation for British anti-lewisite, a drug used against poisoning by lewisite and by some metals; dimercaprol.

balanitis Inflammation of the GLANS PENIS.

balsam Resins combined with oil, applied therapeutically as a soothing agent.

Banti's disease see **splenic anaemia**

barbiturates A group of drugs used as SEDATIVES and in the treatment of insomnia.

barium enema An ENEMA containing barium sulphate, which is opaque to X-RAYS. It is administered in order to outline the lower bowel in RADIOGRAPHY.

barium meal A mixture containing barium sulphate, swallowed by the patient in order to outline the DIGESTIVE TRACT in RADIOGRAPHY.

barotrauma Damage to some part of the body, such as the ear drums or lungs, which has been subjected to abnormal change of pressure, resulting, for example, from the effects of blast or deep-sea diving.

Bartholin's glands Two small lubricating glands, one at each side of the entrance to the vagina.

basal metabolic rate The energy used by the body in a complete state of rest, that is, what is required to maintain life. An abnormally high or low rate may be a feature of disorders of the THYROID GLAND.

Basedow's disease see **thyrotoxicosis**

battered baby syndrome Small children deliberately and repeatedly injured by their parents or guardians. The doctor may be given a false history of accidental injury. (See SYNDROME)

B.C. An abbreviation for bone conduction. (see RINNE TEST)

B.C.G. vaccine Abbreviation for Bacille Calmette-Guérin, Calmette and Guérin being the French scientists who developed the vaccine. It consists of a preparation of live but attenuated TUBERCULOSIS bacilli, which provide immunization against the disease.

beat joint A term applied to INFLAMMATION of an elbow or knee, caused by repeated small blows or sustained pressure. It is mainly an occupational disease, being found, for example, in miners.

bed sore or **decubitus ulcer** INFLAMMATION and ulceration of an area of skin due to prolonged pressure, such as may develop in elderly or weakened patients who lie relatively immobile in bed. Preventive care includes careful nursing, attention to the skin, changing the patients frequently, the application of pads to avoid pressure on the commonly affected parts, e.g. buttocks and heels, and sometimes the use of RIPPLE BEDS or special cushions.

bed wetting see **enuresis**

Behcet's syndrome A condition of POLYARTHRITIS, ULCERS of the mouth and genital region, inflammation of the eyes and of the blood vessels.

Bell's palsy or **facial paralysis** Damage to the nerve controlling the muscles of one side of the face, with their resulting paralysis. The corner of the mouth droops open, wrinkles on one side of the forehead relax and the eye cannot be properly closed. With prompt treatment recovery is generally complete, although in elderly people some weakness may persist.

bends, the This is a popular name for DECOMPRESSION SICKNESS.

benign Describes a relatively mild illness unlikely to worsen or recur. A benign TUMOUR will not disseminate in the body. (Compare MALIGNANT)

Bennett's fracture A fracture at its base of the bone between the thumb and the wrist (the 'first metacarpal'), with some displacement and joint damage.

beri–beri A disease due to lack of vitamin B_1 in the diet. It can cause NEURITIS, with paralysis and loss of feeling, and also heart failure. (See VITAMINS)

Besnier's prurigo A highly irritable form of PRURIGO affecting chiefly the folds of the knees and elbows. As a result of repeated scratching the affected skin tends to become very thickened. The condition is sometimes associated with ALLERGIC conditions like asthma or hay fever.

bezoar A mass of substance swallowed repeatedly but not digested and remaining in the stomach.

biceps A Y-shaped muscle formed of two separate upper parts which unite to make a single muscle. The biceps of the front of the upper arm is an example.

bicuspid 1 A tooth with two points or cusps; one of the premolar teeth. (See TEETH) **2** The mitral valve of the heart. (See HEART)

b.i.d. A prescription indication meaning 'twice a day' – the initials of the Latin words 'bis in die'.

bilateral On both sides.

bile A thick yellow-green digestive juice secreted by the liver. After being stored in the gall bladder it passes into the duodenum where it serves to break down fats in the food and deposit them in an EMULSION form in the intestinal contents. (See DIGESTIVE TRACT)

bile duct The tube taking the bile from the gall bladder to the duodenum. (See DIGESTIVE TRACT)

bilharziasis

bilharziasis see **schistosomiasis**

biliary colic COLIC of the tubes carrying bile from the gall bladder to the duodenum (see DIGESTIVE TRACT). It is due to an obstruction caused by a CALCULUS in one of the tubes.

bilirubin An orange pigment found in BILE.

bilirubinaemia The presence of BILIRUBIN in the blood.

biliuria Presence of BILE in the urine. (See JAUNDICE)

biliverdin A green pigment found in bile.

binaural Relating to both ears.

binocular Relating to both eyes.

biochemistry The science of chemical processes in the living organism.

biofeedback The use of electronic apparatus to monitor by sound or similar signal some of the working of a patient's AUTONOMIC NERVOUS SYSTEM. For instance, tension or raised blood pressure can signal their presence through apparatus attached to the skin of the patient who is then said to be able to control these factors.

biopsy The removal of a small piece of TISSUE from a patient for microscopic examination as an aid to DIAGNOSIS.

birth control The regulation of birth by the prevention or control of conception.

bisexual 1 A hermaphrodite. **2** Sexually attracted to both males and females.

blackhead see **acne**

blackwater fever A rare and severe complication of one form of MALARIA. Pigment produced from the breaking down of RED BLOOD CELLS passes into and discolours the urine, and also damages the kidneys.

bladder see **gall bladder; urinary bladder**

blastomycosis Severe infection caused by a FUNGUS, blastomyces.

bleeding time A simple test to estimate the clotting power of a patient's blood by noting the time required for bleeding from a skin puncture to stop. (See COAGULATION)

blepharitis Inflammation of the eyelid.

blister A raised area of skin holding fluid, generally PLASMA, which has seeped out of underlying blood vessels. A 'blood blister' contains whole blood which has escaped from damaged vessels under skin that is still intact.

block 1 See HEART BLOCK. **2** Local anaesthesia in a part of the body achieved by injecting a fluid to reduce the sensitivity of nerves in that area.

blood An adult has very approximately one pint of blood for each 14 lbs of body weight. Travelling through a closed system of vessels, blood has many functions besides the transport of oxygen and nutrients to the tissues and the removal of waste products. Since it circulates to every part of the body, it is the chemical intercommunication system between all tissues and organs (see LUNGS, LIVER, KIDNEY, HORMONE). The cells it contains play their essential parts (see ERYTHROCYTE, LEUCOCYTES, PLATELETS). By widening and narrowing some of the blood vessels, as at the skin, blood also helps control the body temperature.

blood count A laboratory test to determine the numbers of the different blood cells in each cubic millimetre of a patient's blood.

blood groups Two factors found in the blood have been labelled A and B. Their presence or absence determines the group of the blood: containing A, or B, or both (group AB), or neither (group O). In addition, regardless of its grouping within the A and B system, an individual's blood can contain the RHESUS FACTOR (Rhesus positive) or be without it (Rhesus negative). The presence or absence of these factors has no bearing on health. However, in blood transfusion it is important that a patient does not receive blood carrying a factor which is absent from his own blood. His body would react as if a foreign substance had been injected and would produce ANTIBODIES to cause agglutination of the red cells of his transfused blood. This could make him dangerously ill.

   Before any transfusion great care is taken to check blood groups. This includes cross-matching, a drop of the patient's blood being tested against a sample of the blood to be transfused to ensure that no AGGLUTINATION results.

blood poisoning A layman's term for SEPTICAEMIA or PYAEMIA. It is also sometimes inaccurately used to describe a severe abscess or skin infection.

blood pressure The pressure with which the heart pumps the blood into the arteries. It is measured in millimetres of mercury, i.e. the pressure needed to maintain a column of mercury at given height of millimetres. The measurement is twofold, the higher being the SYSTOLIC, with the heart contracting, and the lower the DIASTOLIC, with the heart relaxing.

blue baby A non-technical term for a baby with a congenital heart defect which prevents the efficient circulation of oxygen-laden blood. With inadequate oxygen the face, especially at the lips and nose, has a blue rather than pink, complexion.

B.M.R. An abbreviation for BASAL METABOLIC RATE.

boil see **furuncle**

bone conduction see **Rinne test**

bone marrow see **marrow**

booster An extra dose of vaccine, given some time after the completion of the original vaccine course, in order to maintain the immunizing effect before it begins to fade.

borborygmus A rumbling noise in the abdomen caused by gas in the bowels.

Bornholm disease or **epidemic pleurodynia** An epidemic VIRUS illness with influenza-like features and, in addition, sharp chest pains. It was first noted on the Danish island of Bornholm.

B.P. An abbreviation for BLOOD PRESSURE.

brachial Relating to the upper arm.

bradycardia A slow pulse rate.

Braille A system of printing representing letters by combinations of raised dots to enable the blind to read by touch.

brain (see pages 36 – 37)

brain stem The lower stem-like portion of the BRAIN, connecting it with the SPINAL CORD.

brain

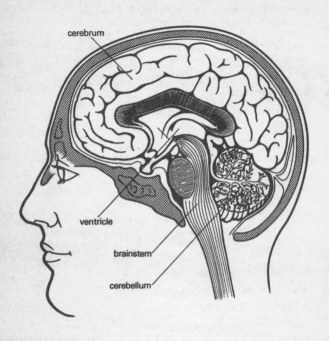

The structure of the brain

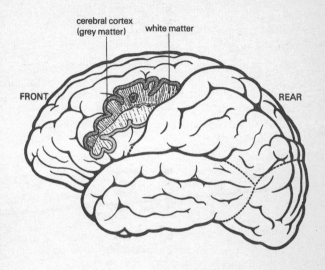

FRONT

REAR

cerebral cortex
(grey matter)

white matter

The brain with part cut away to show the cerebral cortex or grey matter. See also CRANIAL NERVES *for view of lower surface.*

branchial cyst

branchial cyst or **branchial fistula** A CYST or FISTULA on one side of the neck, originating in the persistence of a structure which normally disappears during the development of the FOETUS.

breakbone fever see **dengue**

breath sound The sound of breathing as heard by AUSCULTATION of the chest.

breech delivery The birth of a baby buttocks first instead of the usual VERTEX DELIVERY.

breech presentation Position of the baby in the womb before birth and during DELIVERY, with the buttocks first.

bregma see **fontanelles**

Bright's disease The old name for certain forms of NEPHRITIS.

bronchi (singular, *bronchus*) The air passages branching from the TRACHEA into the lungs. (See LUNGS)

bronchial Relating to the BRONCHI.

bronchiectasis A chronic disease of the BRONCHI and BRONCHIOLES, which lose their elasticity, become permanently enlarged and fill with sticky mucus or pus.

bronchiole One of the smallest branches of the BRONCHI.

bronchitis Inflammation of the BRONCHI.

bronchodilator A drug used to reduce the contracting spasm of BRONCHI, as in ASTHMA.

bronchography X-ray examination of the lungs after introducing into the BRONCHI a preparation opaque to X-rays in order to outline them.

bronchopneumonia Infection of the lungs, generally beginning at the level of the BRONCHIOLES and producing scattered patches of inflammation. (Compare LOBAR PNEUMONIA)

bronchoscope An illuminated tube with optical fittings which is passed down the TRACHEA in order to examine the BRONCHI.

bronchospasm Narrowing of the BRONCHI caused by a spasm of their encircling muscles.

brucellosis A bacterial disease caught from the infected milk of cattle or goats, or through contact with these animals. Symptoms of fever, aching, prostration and sweating come in attacks which may clear up and then recur over many weeks.

bruise An escape of blood under the skin caused by ruptured blood vessels.

bruit A heart MURMUR heard on AUSCULTATION.

bubonic plague see **plague**

buccal Relating to the mouth.

Buerger's disease or **thrombo-angiitis obliterans** This is characterized by a narrowing of blood vessels in the limbs, with inflammation and a tendency to form blood clots. Walking becomes painful and may be limited to quite short distances. There is also risk of gangrene. The disease affects mainly men, and is made much worse by smoking.

bulla A blister.

burns

burns These can be caused by heat, electricity, chemicals and IONIZING RADIATION. Tissues are destroyed and blood vessels in the area become more permeable, plasma oozing out as shown by BLISTERS. If the burn is large this loss of blood fluid can produce SHOCK, which is the immediate danger to the patient. Later dangers are the development of infection and the appearance of disfiguring and handicapping scars.

bursa A fibrous tissue sac containing a small amount of fluid, reducing friction in areas where ligaments move at joints. A bursa may develop at points where abnormal pressure occurs, for example, on the foot, where it is called a bunion.

bursitis Inflammation of a BURSA.

byssinosis PNEUMOCONIOSIS caused by inhalation of cotton dust.

C **cachexia** Severe malnutrition, loss of weight and weakness.

cadaver A dead body, especially one used for anatomical study and dissection.

caecostomy Surgical construction of an artificial opening between the CAECUM and the abdominal wall to permit evacuation of FAECES when the COLON and ANUS cannot be used. (See DIGESTIVE TRACT)

caecum The pouch-like beginning of the large intestine (see DIGESTIVE TRACT). The APPENDIX opens into it.

Caesarean section Delivery of a baby through the abdominal wall and UTERUS by surgical operation.

Caisson disease see **decompression sickness**

calcaneus or **os calcis** The bone at the heel of the foot.

calcification Formation of deposits of calcium salts in a tissue.

calculus (plural, *calculi*) An abnormal hard deposit formed and lying loose in a hollow organ; a stone. The common sites are the kidney and the gall bladder but calculi can also be found in the urinary bladder, having moved there from the kidney, and in such organs as the PROSTATE GLAND or the SALIVARY GLANDS. Calculi may present no symptoms unless they cause pressure by size and number, or give rise to bleeding or to colic by obstructing a duct.

caliper A special splint worn by a patient, which is designed to protect and strengthen damaged or weakened bone or muscle.

callosity A hardened, thickened and raised area of skin, generally formed as a result of sustained pressure or rubbing.

callus 1 A CALLOSITY. **2** A hard material that develops around broken bone and within which new bone will form.

calorie A unit of heat. The small or gram calorie (c) is the quantity of heat required to raise the temperature of one gram of water by one degree centigrade. The large or kilogram calorie (C) is the quantity of heat required to raise the temperature of one kilogram of water by one-degree centigrade. The kilogram calorie is used in dietetics to calculate the energy value in food.

cancellous bone The lighter, more porous bone tissue which lies within the outer COMPACT BONE.

cancer A malignant tumour.

cancrum oris Severe infection of the mouth with gangrene.

Candida see **Monilia**

candidiasis or **candidosis** Infection with MONILIA.

canine teeth see **teeth**

cannula A metal tube inserted into a body cavity to introduce or remove fluid.

canthus The corner of each side of the eye where the upper and lower lids meet.

capillaries The smallest blood vessels in the body, forming a fine network in all tissues. They provide the cells with nutrients. (See CIRCULATION OF THE BLOOD)

capitate One of the small CARPAL BONES. (See SKELETON)

carbohydrates Energy- and heat-producing substances which are high in calories. Starches and sugars are carbohydrate foods.

carbon dioxide A colourless, odourless gas, present in air in small amounts. It is produced by the life processes of the body and exhaled through the lungs. (See CIRCULATION OF THE BLOOD)

carbon monoxide A colourless, odourless gas which is poisonous to the body since it interferes with the carrying of oxygen by the blood. It is present in the exhaust fumes of cars and in fires with incomplete combustion caused by poor ventilation.

carbuncle An infection of the skin formed by a spreading FURUNCLE or a close group of several furuncles.

carcinogen A substance which can produce CANCER.

carcinoma A CANCER which arises in the skin or in lining membranes, e.g., of the intestinal tract. (Compare SARCOMA)

cardiac Relating to the HEART.

cardiac asthma A sudden attack of breathlessness with severe CONGESTION of the lungs caused by ACUTE heart failure. It has no connection with the ordinary or bronchial ASTHMA.

cardiac catheterization The passage of a thin CATHETER through a vein of the arm or neck into the HEART. This allows direct study of pressure changes, the collection of blood samples and the X-raying of changes within the heart.

cardiac compression or **cardiac massage** see **heart massage**

cardiology The study of the heart and its diseases.

cardiovascular Relating to the heart and the blood vessels.

cardioversion The use of electrical apparatus to correct some forms of abnormal heart beat rhythm. (See also DEFIBRILLATION)

caries Decay, especially of teeth or bones.

carminative A medicine prescribed to relieve FLATULENCE by making the patient belch.

carotenaemia An excessive amount of the pigment carotene in the blood, giving a yellow tinge to the skin; a form of XANTHOSIS.

carpal

carpal Relating to the wrist and to the bones which comprise it.

carpal tunnel syndrome Pain, numbness and tingling in the fingers, and weakness of the thumb. This occurs when a nerve which passes to the palm of the hand through the 'carpal tunnel' of bones and fibrous bands at the wrist becomes compressed within the tunnel.

carpo–pedal spasm A spasm of muscles in which the hands and feet go into forced flexion. (See also TETANY)

carrier Someone who can, unharmed, carry in his body infectious BACTERIA which he may unknowingly pass on to others who are susceptible to them.

cartilage A thick white fibrous TISSUE; gristle. It is found at the end of bone shafts, where it forms smooth surfaces for the movement of joints, or in firm pliable areas like the ear, or as cushioning pads like the INTERVERTEBRAL DISC or the MENISCUS of the knee.

castration Surgical removal of the TESTICLES and the consequent reduction of male sexual characteristics.

C.A.T. An abbreviation for COMPUTERIZED AXIAL TOMOGRAPHY.

catabolism The process by which complex chemical substances are broken down in the body into simpler ones. (Compare ANABOLISM)

catalepsy A trance-like state in which the patient assumes an immobile posture. The cause is emotional.

cataract A condition in which part or the whole of the lens of the EYE becomes opaque, impairing vision.

catarrh Inflammation of any MUCOUS MEMBRANE in the body, with a great increase of its normal MUCUS discharge. The term is commonly used to mean inflammation of the membranes of nose and throat. (See RHINITIS, SINUSITIS)

catatonia A condition occasionally found in SCHIZOPHRENIA in which the patient appears out of touch with his surroundings, reacting with purposeless excitement (sometimes violence) or meaningless repetitive gestures and speech, or displaying a trance-like state of immobility.

catgut Material used in a SUTURE. Made from the intestines of the sheep, it is slowly absorbed by the body after the wound has healed.

catharsis see **abreaction**

catheter A tube which is passed through body passages into a normal body cavity in order to introduce or remove fluids, as, for example, a catheter passed through the URETHRA to extract urine from the bladder.

cat-scratch fever A virus infection which can be caught from the scratch or bite of a cat. After an INCUBATION PERIOD of one to three weeks the patient shows fever and enlargement of the LYMPH GLANDS.

caudal Towards the lower end of the human body or, in an animal, towards the tail.

causalgia A severe burning pain caused by injury to a nerve.

cauterize To destroy or burn TISSUE by the controlled application of heat, electricity, laser beams or a suitable chemical. Cauterization is also used to stop bleeding in small blood vessels by COAGULATION and to stimulate the repair of damaged tissues.

cavernous haemangioma A tumour of CONNECTIVE TISSUE with many enclosed spaces containing blood.

cc and **ccm** Abbreviations for cubic centimetre (liquid measure).

C.D.H. An abbreviation for CONGENITAL DISCLOCATION OF THE HIP.

cell The smallest entity capable of life within all living things and the basic unit of the human body. Each microscopic cell has an outer membrane, and is filled with jellylike cytoplasm within which lie the nucleus and other minute structures. The TISSUES of the body are made of agglomerations of their own characteristic cells.

cellular tissue A type of connective tissue which by its loose texture allows some movement between the tissues attached to either side of it, for example, between the skin and the underlying structures.

cellulitis Inflammation of CELLULAR TISSUE. The term is generally applied to a spreading infection in the loose tissue beneath the skin.

celsius see **centigrade**

cement or **cementum** A thin bone-like layer covering the roots of teeth, helping to fix them in position.

centigrade A measurement of degree of temperature, shown as °C. It depends on a scale of equal degrees between 0°C for the melting point of ice and 100°C for the boiling point of water. The normal body temperature of a human being is given as 37°C but can range slightly above or below this.

central nervous system The BRAIN and the SPINAL CORD.

cephalalgia A headache.

cerebellum A large part of the BRAIN, filling the rear part of the skull. Its main function is the coordination of muscle action and the maintenance of balance.

cerebral Relating to the brain.

cerebral cortex The outer coating of grey matter of the brain, with layers of nerve cells.

cerebral palsy The medical term for 'spastic', it is used to describe failure of development of, or damage to, some part of the brain. Cerebral palsy can arise during pregnancy or labour or in the course of a severe illness shortly after birth, but it is not HEREDITARY. The consequences vary according to the part of the brain affected. SPASTIC muscles, ATHETOSIS and ATAXIA are common but there may be no signs until retarded activity and abnormal movements are noted as the baby develops. Other possible handicaps involve vision, speech, hearing and the sense of touch. Mental backwardness and EPILEPSY are also common.

cerebration The working activity of the brain.

cerebrospinal fever see **meningococcal meningitis**

cerebrospinal fluid A clear fluid which surrounds the BRAIN and SPINAL CORD in the subarachnoid space (see MENINGES) and fills the ventricles of the brain and the thin central canal of the SPINAL CORD.

cerebrovascular Relating to the blood vessels of the
  BRAIN.

cerebrovascular accident see **stroke**

cerebrum The largest and uppermost part of the BRAIN,
  consisting of the two cerebral hemispheres.

cerumen The wax which forms in the ear canal.

cervical 1 Relating to the neck. **2** Relating to the CERVIX.

cervical cap A small cupped rubber contraceptive. It is
  fitted over the CERVIX before intercourse to cover the
  opening of the womb.

cervical rib A small and sometimes rudimentary rib,
  additional to the normal number in the body, which is
  attached to the lowest cervical VERTEBRA. Its presence
  may cause pain or discomfort in the arm resulting from
  pressure on blood vessels and nerves.

cervical smear A simple routine examination of cells from
  the CERVIX to ascertain whether it carries any immediate
  or future danger of cancer.

cervicitis Inflammation at the neck of the womb. (See
  REPRODUCTIVE SYSTEM, FEMALE)

cervix The neck-like entrance to the womb. (See
  REPRODUCTIVE SYSTEM, FEMALE)

Chagas' disease A parasitic infestation by a form of
  TRYPANOSOME found in South America and transmitted
  to man by an insect. The MICRO-ORGANISMS pass through
  the patient's blood to the heart muscle and to the digestive
  system. The disease may cause sudden heart failure.

chancre The first sore of SYPHILIS at the site of entry of
  infection, e.g. genitals or mouth. It may appear as a hard

painless spot of inflammation which then resolves while the infection settles deeper in the body.

chancroid A soft open sore on the genitals – a VENEREAL DISEASE not related to SYPHILIS – caused by infection with bacteria called Haemophilus ducreyi.

cheilitis Inflammation of the lips.

cheilosis Cracks and dry scaling of the lips and at the corners of the mouth. The condition is sometimes associated with a deficiency of RIBOFLAVIN.

chelating agent A chemical which will combine with certain metals, used in cases of poisoning with these metals to render them harmless.

chemosis Swelling of the CONJUNCTIVA.

chemotherapy Treatment of infections with drugs, including ANTIBIOTICS, which damage MICRO-ORGANISMS.

Cheyne–Stokes respiration A pattern of irregular breathing in which respiration is in cycles; at first slow, shallow and slight and increasing gradually in depth and speed until it fades again, appears to stop and then resumes. It is present in some serious conditions associated with a disturbance of the brain's centre for controlling breathing.

chicken pox A virus infection, with a rash, commonly occurring in epidemics in children. The medical name is varicella. (See FEVERS OF CHILDHOOD)

chigger The name given to various types of small insect found in hot climates, which irritate the skin by biting or burrowing into it.

chilblains A reaction of the skin to excessive cold, the superficial blood vessels being greatly restricted, producing patches of redness and swelling, with itching and burning. The extremities, such as feet, hands, nose and ears, are especially affected.

chiropody The study of the foot and the treatment of its diseases.

chiropractic A non-medical method of treatment, mainly by manipulation of the bones, especially of the VERTEBRAE. It is based on the concept that many diseases are due to a displacement of the bones which produces pressure on the nerves.

choking Interruption of breathing by obstruction of the air entry into the lungs. The obstruction may be external, a covering over nose and mouth, heavy smoke, or a cord compressing the neck. It may be internal, as when heavy smoke, mud, food or vomit block the TRACHEA.

chol- A prefix meaning 'relating to BILE.'

cholangitis Inflammation of the tubes leading the BILE from the GALL BLADDER to the DUODENUM.

cholecyst- A prefix meaning 'relating to the GALL BLADDER.'

cholecystectomy Surgical removal of the GALL BLADDER.

cholecystitis INFLAMMATION of the GALL BLADDER.

cholecystogram An X-ray picture of the GALL BLADDER. This is generally taken after injecting into the patient's veins a substance opaque to X-rays which collects in the gall bladder.

cholelithiasis Stones in the GALL BLADDER.

cholera A severe disease caught from food or water contaminated with infected FAECES. A BACTERIUM, vibrio cholerae, multiplies in the intestines and causes intense watery DIARRHOEA. The patient suffers from marked DEHYDRATION, with loss of important body salts, painful cramps and prostration.

cholesteatoma A mass formed by surface sheddings of skin or skin growth from the outer ear pressing inwards through a perforated eardrum into the middle ear. (See EAR)

cholesterol A fat-like chemical found in some foods and in most parts of the body. It is a major component of the ATHEROMA.

chondritis Inflammation of CARTILAGE.

chondro– A prefix meaning 'relating to CARTILAGE'.

chondroma A BENIGN TUMOUR of CARTILAGE.

chondrosarcoma A MALIGNANT TUMOUR of CARTILAGE.

chordee A painful curved erection of the penis.

chorea A nervous disorder causing constant muscle spasms with involuntary, jerky movements of the limbs and twitching of the face. HUNTINGDON'S CHOREA and SYDENHAM'S CHOREA are two quite unrelated forms.

chorion The outer of the two membranes which surround the developing FOETUS in the womb.

choroid The middle one of the three layers forming the wall of the eyeball. (See EYE)

choroid plexus A network of small blood vessels inside the ventricles of the BRAIN. They secrete the CEREBRO–SPINAL FLUID.

Christmas disease A blood disease in which COAGULATION is defective and bleeding readily occurs.

chromosome One of the minute particles formed from the NUCLEUS when a CELL divides. They carry the GENES which determine the inherited characteristics of the new cells. In human cells the chromosomes number 46, arranged in 23 pairs. One pair relates to the sex of the individual to whom the cell belongs. In the female this pair consists of two X chromosomes. In the male it has one X and one Y chromosome.

chronic A term used to describe an illness of slow onset and long duration. The opposite is ACUTE.

chyle A milky fluid in the lymph vessels containing an EMULSION of fat absorbed from food.

chyme An almost liquid mass of partly digested food which passes from the stomach to the intestine.

cicatrix A scar.

cilia Short microscopic hair-like processes projecting from the cells lining some body passages. Their movements help small particles to be swept away. Cilia within the air passages, for example, propel dust or MUCUS upwards.

circulation of the blood This is the continuous movement of BLOOD from the HEART through ARTERIES, CAPILLARIES and VEINS back to the heart. There are in fact two principal circulations, one to bring oxygen to the tissues and the other to carry blood to the lungs to be replenished with oxygen. (see opposite)

Diagrammatically, the left side of the heart pumps oxygen-rich blood into the arteries which divide into smaller and smaller branches until at each microscopic

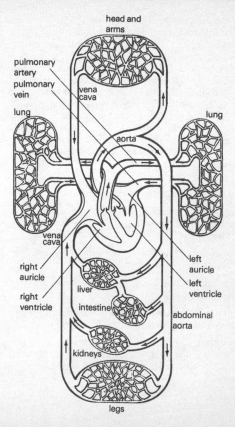

head and
arms

pulmonary
artery

pulmonary
vein

vena
cava

lung

aorta

lung

vena
cava

right
auricle

right
ventricle

liver

intestine

kidneys

left
auricle

left
ventricle

abdominal
aorta

legs

circulation of the blood

tissue site they form a network of microscopic vessels, the capillaries. Here oxygen and other nutritional matter pass to the cells. From the cells carbon dioxide and other waste materials pass into the blood. From the capillaries small veins lead the blood back towards the heart, being joined by other veins until large veins bring the blood back to the right side of the heart. This pumps it to the lungs by a similar, if smaller, system of arteries, capillaries and veins. At the lung capillaries fresh oxygen is taken into the blood, and carbon dioxide is given out to escape in the exhaled air. The circulation is complete when the blood returns to the left side of the heart to resume its circular tour.

circumcision Surgical removal of part of the loose foreskin which covers the end of the PENIS.

cirrhosis A condition in which, as a result of inflammation, the tissues of the liver become hard and fibrous.

claudication A medical term for limping. (See also INTERMITTENT CLAUDICATION)

claustrophobia Fear of being in a confined or crowded space or a small room.

clavicle The bone which joins the shoulder to the sternum or breastbone; the collarbone. (See SKELETON)

cleft palate A congenital defect producing a fissure or opening in the PALATE, thus connecting the cavities of the mouth and nose. It can be repaired by means of plastic surgery.

climacteric see **menopause**

clinical Relating to the findings by a doctor about a patient in bed or on an examination couch, as opposed to special investigations using laboratory or X-ray methods.

clitoris A small elongated body at the front of the VULVA, sensitive in sexual activity when stimulated by friction.

clonus Involuntary rapidly alternating contraction and relaxation of muscle.

clotting see **coagulation**

clubbing Medical term for thickening and broadening of the tips of fingers and toes, associated with CHRONIC diseases which impair respiration.

club foot A deformity of the foot which is turned inwards or outwards at the ankle. It is generally CONGENITAL.

C.N.S. An abbreviation for CENTRAL NERVOUS SYSTEM.

coagulation The clotting process of blood, which controls bleeding from a cut vessel. It depends on a complicated inter-reaction of many chemicals and of PLATELETS, and on the formation of fibrin – threads of PROTEIN which make the clot by enmeshing the blood. Clots may also form in uncut vessels. (See THROMBUS)

coarctation A narrowing or stricture. The term is generally used with reference to the AORTA.

cocci see under **bacteria**

coccydynia Pain in the region of the COCCYX, due generally to injury of that bone.

coccyx A small triangular bone which forms the lower end of the backbone.

cochlea A spiral cavity within the ear containing the main organ for receiving sound. (See EAR)

coeliac disease A disease in young children caused by inability to digest and assimilate some foods, especially fats. Loss of weight, a swollen abdomen, and severe DIARRHOEA with pale STOOLS, are characteristic features. The condition is associated with a hypersensitivity to GLUTEN, which must be eliminated from the diet.

coitus Sexual intercourse.

coitus interruptus During sexual intercourse the withdrawal of the penis before orgasm in an attempt to avoid conception. It is a generally unreliable method.

cold see **common cold**

cold sore see **herpes simplex**

colic 1 Waves of pain arising from inflammation or obstruction of a hollow organ. They are caused by distension and strong constriction of the involuntary MUSCLES of the organ. Colicky pain tends to make the sufferer move and writhe rather than lie still. **2** A popular term for the digestive discomforts of small babies.

coliform A group of bacteria, one species of which is a normal COMMENSAL in the bowel, but which can cause infection in other parts of the body, such as the bladder and kidneys. Other species cause intestinal illnesses.

colitis Inflammation of the COLON. (See also ULCERATIVE COLITIS)

collagen A PROTEIN which forms an important part of the CONNECTIVE TISSUE.

collagen diseases Several types of disease causing INFLAMMATION of CONNECTIVE TISSUE. Some skin conditions and some forms of rheumatism are examples.

collarbone see **clavicle**

Colles' fracture Fracture of one or both of the bones of the forearm immediately above the wrist.

colon The large intestine, extending from the CAECUM to the RECTUM. (See DIGESTIVE TRACT)

colostomy Surgical construction of an artificial opening between the colon and abdominal wall to permit evacuation of FAECES when the anus cannot be used. (See DIGESTIVE TRACT)

colostrum A thin clear fluid secreted by the breasts in the first few days after childbirth, subsequently replaced by milk.

colour blindness Inability to distinguish clearly between certain colours, a congenital condition found mostly in men. Difficulty in telling red from green is the most common form.

colpo- A prefix meaning 'relating to the vagina.'

colporrhaphy The operation of suturing the vagina, e.g., in the treatment of PROLAPSE of the uterus.

coma Deep unconsciousness from which a patient cannot be roused.

comedo or **comedone** see **acne**

commensal A plant or animal which lives on or within the body without harming it, such as some bacteria which are normally present in the intestine. (Compare PARASITE)

comminuted fracture A fracture in which the broken part of the bone is in several separate small pieces.

common cold Acute inflammation of the MUCOUS MEMBRANE lining the nose and throat. It is due to a VIRUS infection and may be worsened by SECONDARY infection from bacteria.

compact bone The dense, hard bone tissue which forms in the outer layer of bones.

complex A group of ideas or beliefs arising subconsciously from forgotten or repressed experiences in the past, but powerfully affecting and directing behaviour. (See also REPRESSION)

compress A folded cloth or pad heated or soaked in cold or hot fluid and applied to the skin to ease pain or improve circulation in the area.

computerized axial tomography A form of TOMOGRAPHY by which images can be made of a whole plane or cross-section across a selected part of the body.

conception 1 Union of the male SPERMATOZOON with the female OVUM; fertilization. **2** The beginning of pregnancy.

concussion A jarring of the brain caused by a blow to the head and resulting in immediate unconsciousness. Recovery is generally well within 24 hours and is likely to be complete unless there are additional injuries to the skull or brain.

conditioned reflex An involuntary or automatic bodily or emotional reaction to some originally unconnected stimulus. The response has developed as a result of association or experience. An example would be mouth watering or hunger at the sound of a bell which had been repeatedly used to announce meal times. Much of the motorist's handling of his car controls in traffic is related to conditioned reflexes.

condom A thin rubber sheath worn over the penis during intercourse to prevent conception or infection.

condyle A rounded end found in some bones, generally where they form a JOINT with another bone.

congenital Present or occurring at the time of birth but not necessarily HEREDITARY.

congenital dislocation of the hip A rare condition at birth in which the baby has slack ligaments at the hip joint, so that the FEMUR slips out of its position in the socket at the PELVIS. If diagnosed early this is easily corrected by temporary splinting.

congestion Abnormal and excessive accumulation of blood in the blood vessels of an organ.

conjunctiva The thin membrane which covers the eyeball and the inside surfaces of the eyelids.

conjunctivitis Inflammation of the CONJUNCTIVA; 'pink eye' or 'red eye'.

connective tissue Relatively less specialized TISSUE which binds together or provides filling between other tissues in the body. It may be fatty or fibrous in texture.

constipation Inability, infrequency or difficulty in passing motions. There is no 'normal' frequency, since bowel action depends greatly on habit and diet. Delayed evacuation of the bowel is in itself harmless and painless, and purgatives should be avoided unless medically prescribed. The aim should be to regularize habit.

consumption An old term for any wasting disease, especially TUBERCULOSIS of the lungs.

contact dermatitis Acute DERMATITIS caused by contact of the skin with a substance to which the patient is sensitive.

contact lens Glass or plastic lenses worn instead of spectacles, fitting directly on the front of the eyeball and almost invisible in wear.

contagious disease An infection which can be transmitted by direct contact with the infected person, his body secretions, his belongings or things that have been handled by him.

contraception see **birth control**

contralateral On the side of the body opposite to the position of something already referred to.

contrast medium A liquid opaque to X-rays which is passed into a body tube or cavity to outline its shape in RADIOGRAPHY.

contrecoup The injurious effect on one side of the brain of a blow received on the opposite side of the skull.

controls In experimental studies or evaluations of treatment the controls are those cases not undergoing the experiments or treatments in question, and against which the results can be compared.

contusion An injury or bruising on some part of the body which leaves the skin intact.

convulsion An involuntary, rapidly alternating contraction and relaxation of muscles, generally accompanied by unconsciousness; a fit.

Cooley's anaemia see **thalassaemia**

Coomb's test A test which is used on the blood for the detection of ERYTHROBLASTOSIS FOETALIS.

copulation Sexual intercourse.

corn A small area of hard, thickened skin, generally on the feet and toes, caused by rubbing or pressure.

cornea The transparent front outer part of the eyeball. (See EYE)

coronary arteries The arteries which provide the heart muscle with its own blood supply.

coronary thrombosis or **coronary occlusion** The blockage of a CORONARY ARTERY by a blood clot. Cessation of blood supply to part of the heart muscle can cause intense pain and SHOCK and failure of the heart.

cor pulmonale A weakness of the heart caused by some chronic diseases of the lungs and their blood vessels.

corpus luteum A small yellow mass at the surface of the OVARY, formed at the point where an OVUM is released. If CONCEPTION follows it secretes HORMONES to protect the pregnancy. Otherwise it atrophies and menstruation follows.

corticosteroids The general name for hormones secreted by the ADRENAL GLAND and also for similar chemicals synthetically made.

corticotrophin A HORMONE secreted by the anterior part of the PITUITARY GLAND. It stimulates the ADRENAL GLAND to produce a CORTICOSTEROID.

coryza The common cold, especially when accompanied by much nasal discharge.

costal Relating to the ribs.

costive Suffering from constipation.

cot death Sudden, unexpected death of an infant who had previously appeared well.

couching A surgical technique which displaces without removing a CATARACT lens so as to allow light to enter the eye.

counterirritant An agent such as a heat liniment or poultice which is applied to the skin to increase local blood supply, induce congestion and relieve pain in underlying organs.

cowpox A virus infection of cattle. It is used in the preparation of vaccine against SMALLPOX since it can give immunity to that disease.

Coxsackie The name of a group of viruses producing a variety of diseases including a form of MENINGITIS and BORNHOLM DISEASE.

cramp A painful and lasting muscle contraction. Its causes include poor blood supply to the muscle or marked salt loss from the body, as with the fluid in heavy sweating or diarrhoea.

cranial nerves The twelve major nerves which arise from the BRAIN. They are numbered as well as named. (see opposite)

craniotomy Surgical opening of the skull, generally for operation on the BRAIN.

cranium That part of the skull which encloses the brain.

crepitus 1 A crackling sound in inflamed lungs heard on AUSCULTATION as the patient breathes. **2** A sensation of

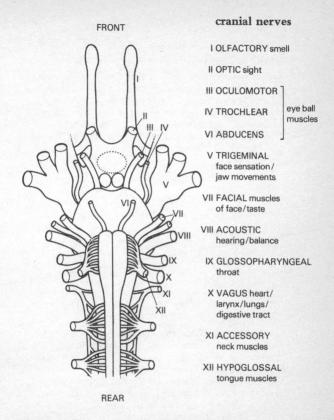

FRONT

cranial nerves

I OLFACTORY smell

II OPTIC sight

III OCULOMOTOR ⌉

IV TROCHLEAR | eye ball
muscles

VI ABDUCENS ⌋

V TRIGEMINAL
face sensation /
jaw movements

VII FACIAL muscles
of face/taste

VIII ACOUSTIC
hearing/balance

IX GLOSSOPHARYNGEAL
throat

X VAGUS heart/
larynx/lungs/
digestive tract

XI ACCESSORY
neck muscles

XII HYPOGLOSSAL
tongue muscles

REAR

*The lower surface of the brain showing the cranial nerves and
listing their main destinations and functions.*

grating felt in the movement of a joint with irregular, rough bone surfaces, or in the ends of a broken bone.

cretin A child born with a deficiency or absence of thyroid gland hormone. As the child grows he is seen to be unusually sleepy and inactive and is slow to put on weight. Eventually (if untreated) he develops a squat body with a pot belly and a thick dry skin, and is mentally retarded. Response to treatment with thyroid is good provided it is begun early.

crisis The sudden change for the better (generally) or the worse in a fever or disease. (Compare LYSIS)

Crohn's disease see **regional enteritis**

cross-matching see **blood groups**

croup Noisy, hoarse, difficult breathing accompanied by a harsh cough, caused by an infection, spasm or thick discharge in the upper air passages and the LARYNX.

crown The upper part of the tooth, above the gum.

cryotherapy The use of cold as a form of treatment, as, for example, the application of carbon dioxide snow to warts in order to remove them.

cryptorchism In the developing male foetus failure of the TESTICLE to move from its original position in the abdomen down into the SCROTUM. This is also described as a maldescended or undescended TESTIS. If the condition does not correct itself spontaneously in the child after birth it may need treatment. The relatively cooler position in the scrotum is necessary for the production of active SPERMATOZOA.

C.S.F. An abbreviation for CEREBROSPINAL FLUID.

cubital Relating to the elbow.

cuboid One of the TARSAL bones. (See SKELETON)

culture The artificial growth of MICRO-ORGANISMS or TISSUE CELLS in the laboratory. The culture medium is the nutrient preparation used for this.

cuneiform The name given to three of the TARSAL bones. (See SKELETON)

cunnilingus In sexual activity oral stimulation of the female genitals.

curette A slim, elongated spoon-shaped surgical instrument used for scraping the internal surface of a hollow organ. (See DILATATION AND CURETTAGE)

cushingoid Having the features of CUSHING'S SYNDROME.

Cushing's syndrome Marked bodily changes due to an excess of CORTICOSTEROIDS. These include water retention, obesity of the trunk, a round ('moon') face, fatigue and muscle weakness, raised blood pressure and, in women, cessation of menstruation. The excess may be due to over-production by the ADRENAL GLAND or to abnormally high secretion of CORTICOTROPHIN by the PITUITARY GLAND. When prolonged treatment of some illnesses by CORTICOSTEROIDS is necessary, this may produce a similar result in the patient.

cutaneous Relating to the skin.

C.V.A. An abbreviation for CEREBRO-VASCULAR ACCIDENT.

cyanocobalamin Vitamin B_{12}. (See VITAMINS)

cyanosis A blue complexion, especially at the lips, nose and ears, caused by an inadequate amount of oxygen in the blood.

cyclitis

cyclitis Inflammation in the eye of the tissues around the IRIS.

cyclothymia A condition of alternating moods of depression and elation.

cyst Any abnormal swelling containing a fluid or jelly-like material, held in place by a sac-like cover.

cystic Relating to or resembling a cyst.

cysticercus A larval form of the TAPEWORM. It can settle in various parts of the body.

cystic fibrosis see **fibrocystic disease**

cystitis Inflammation of the bladder, generally as a result of infection.

cystocoele Protrusion of part of the bladder into the VAGINA.

cystoscope A thin tube-like optical instrument with a light used for inspecting the inside of the bladder after passing through the urethra.

cytology The study of tissues and their cells.

cytotoxic Tending to reduce or suppress the division and reproduction of CELLS. Cytotoxic drugs are used to counteract some forms of cancer, since cancer cells are far more easily affected by them than by ordinary tissue cells.

D **Da Costa's syndrome** or **disordered action of the heart** A condition of anxiety in a patient who develops PALPITATIONS and varied, indefinite chest SYMPTOMS because he fears, quite wrongly, that his heart is diseased. Also called EFFORT SYNDROME.

dacryo- A prefix meaning 'relating to tear fluid' or 'to the tear fluid system of the EYE.' (See also LACRIMAL SYSTEM)

dacryoadenitis Inflammation of the LACRIMAL GLAND.

dacryocystitis Inflammation of the LACRIMAL sac, which is part of the duct system draining the tear fluid to the nose.

D.A.H. An abbreviation for DISORDERED ACTION OF THE HEART. (See DA COSTA'S SYNDROME)

daltonism COLOUR BLINDNESS involving red and green.

D & C An abbreviation for DILATATION AND CURETTAGE.

D & V An abbreviation for 'diarrhoea and vomiting'.

dandruff The small scales of dead skin constantly shed, normally unnoticed, from healthy skin, showing up on the scalp only if their amount is excessive.

deafness Loss of hearing can be caused by trouble in any part of the sound collecting system (see EAR). In the outer ear it can be brought about by blockage of the canal, as by wax, or by damage to the eardrum. In the middle ear deafness can be caused by infection (OTITIS MEDIA), abnormal bone formation at the ossicles or by inflammation or blockage of the EUSTACHIAN CANAL. In the inner ear it can be caused by inflammation of or damage to the COCHLEA or AUDITORY NERVE. Deafness is also classified as *conductive* when the cause is in the ear canal or in the middle ear, and *perceptive* when the cause is in the inner ear or its nerve pathways.

debridement Removal of damaged and dead tissues from a wound to facilitate healing.

decalcification Loss of calcium salts from the bones or teeth, with consequent weakening of their structure.

decompression sickness or **Caisson disease** This results from a sudden reduction in atmospheric pressure and is characterized by many severe symptoms, including pains in the joints ('the bends'), headache, dizziness, paralysis and sometimes even death. It can happen to divers at great depths or to workers in high-pressure chambers (caissons), who breathe in pressurized air, the gases of which tend to dissolve in the blood. If the return to normal pressure is not carried out in carefully graduated stages, the gases come out of solution as bubbles which fill the tissues, giving rise to the symptoms described above. Treatment is by immediate recompression followed by slow decompression.

decongestant A medicine which reduces swelling or CONGESTION.

decubitus The position of a patient lying in bed.

decubitus ulcer see **bed sore**

deep vein thrombosis THROMBOSIS in one of the inner veins of the leg.

defecation Evacuation of the bowels.

defibrillation The restoration of a regular beat to a heart which has VENTRICULAR FIBRILLATION.

defibrillator An apparatus which conveys electrical impulses to the heart to bring about DEFIBRILLATION.

defloration Rupture of the HYMEN.

dehydration Abnormal reduction of water in the body as after severe diarrhoea, vomiting or sweating.

déjà vu The impression that what one is in fact experiencing for the first time is a repetition of a past experience.

Delhi boil see **Leishmaniasis**

delirium A state of mental confusion characterized by excitement and restlessness, often with HALLUCINATIONS and disorientation

delirium tremens A state of delirium which may develop in cases of severe alcoholism.

delivery The act of giving birth to a child.

delusion A firm and unreasonable belief which is not based on reality and which cannot be removed by any demonstration of its inaccuracy.

dementia A condition of CHRONIC or permanent mental deterioration. It is generally used to describe loss of intellectual ability and memory.

dementia paralytica see **general paralysis of the insane**

dementia praecox A former term for SCHIZOPHRENIA.

demyelinating Destroying or reducing the MYELIN sheath of nerve fibres.

dengue or **breakbone fever** A virus disease of the tropics transmitted through mosquito bites. Symptoms include fever, sore throat, headache and very severe pains in the joints.

dentine A very hard substance which forms the main structure of teeth.

deoxyribonucleic acid A very long and complex molecule which, together with protein, forms the CHROMOSOMES. The DNA of each cell carries its specific patterns, a genetic code which is passed on when the cell divides.

depilatory A preparation used on the skin for removing unwanted hair.

depression A state of melancholy abnormal both in depth and duration. 'Reactive depression' follows some calamity which could justifiably cause sadness but occurs with unjustifiable severity. 'Endogenous depression' arises for no obvious reason.

Dercum's disease see **adiposis dolorosa**

dermatitis Inflammation of the skin. (See also ECZEMA)

dermatitis artefacta Skin injuries, such as sores or blisters, deliberately produced by a patient.

dermatographia The raising of a weal on the skin after this has been stroked firmly, a reaction in some cases of ALLERGY.

dermatology The study of the skin and its diseases.

dermatophyte Any microscopic fungus which is capable of invading and infecting the skin, such as TINEA.

dermis The deeper layer of the skin, containing the skin's nerve endings, SEBACEOUS GLANDS, blood vessels and HAIR FOLLICLES. (Compare EPIDERMIS)

dermoid cyst 1 A cyst formed of skin tissue and lying just under the skin. It happens either because of a minor development defect or because a skin fragment has been displaced deep under the surface by accident. **2** A rare cyst formed in the ovary: a TUMOUR of several forms of tissue, generally BENIGN.

desensitization 1 The treatment of an ALLERGIC sensitivity by injecting the patient with a series of small, but gradually increasing doses of the substance to which he is sensitive, so that his body becomes accustomed and immune to it. **2** In psychiatry the treatment of an anxiety or PHOBIA by carefully and repeatedly subjecting the patient to situations which upset him, or by asking him to imagine them. He is taught to relax as this happens, and may be helped by sedatives. Gradually he learns to face these situations without anxiety.

desquamation The shedding of the outer layer of flakes of dead skin, a normal process which, in some skin conditions, can happen to excess.

detached retina see **retinal detachment**

devil's grip see **Bornholm disease**

dextro– A prefix meaning 'on the right side'.

dextrocardia A congenital condition in which the heart is situated towards the right instead of the left side of the chest. In itself it has no detrimental effect on health. (See also SITUS INVERSUS)

dhobie itch 1 CONTACT DERMATITIS caused by marking-ink used on clothes by Indian laundrymen. **2** Infection by TINEA of the skin of the groin.

diabetes insipidus A rare disease in which the patient passes abnormally large amounts of urine. It is caused by the failure of the PITUITARY GLAND to secrete a HORMONE which regulates the activity of the kidneys. It bears no relation to DIABETES MELLITUS.

diabetes mellitus Generally referred to simply as diabetes, this is a disease in which the level of sugar in the blood rises above the normal as a result of inadequate INSULIN secretion by the PANCREAS or the body's inability to use the insulin secreted.

diadochokinesis The ability to stop one set of muscle actions and substitute an exactly opposite set, for example, the rapid turning of the hand and forearm back and forth in opposite directions. This is used as a test of the integrity of some parts of the nervous system.

diagnosis The doctor's decision as to the exact nature of his patient's illness. This may involve four main features. **1** The history; how the illness developed. **2** The symptoms: what the patient feels and notices. **3** The signs: what the doctor finds on methodical examination of the patient. **4** Investigations: the result of special tests, for example, on the blood or by X-ray.

dialysis The use of a special semi-permeable membrane to extract from a liquid substances which will filter through it. This principle is employed in the KIDNEY MACHINE.

diaphoresis Perspiration, especially excessive perspiration.

diaphragm 1 A large dome-shaped fibrous and muscular sheet separating the chest cavity from the abdominal cavity. Its movements play a major part in respiration by allowing the lungs to expand and contract, drawing in and expelling air. **2** A dome-shaped rubber or plastic contraceptive; the Dutch cap. It is inserted in the vagina before intercourse and covers the opening of the womb.

diaphysis The shaft of a long bone. (Compare EPIPHYSIS)

diarrhoea The frequent passing of loose, watery stools.

diastole The phase in each heart beat when the VENTRICLES are relaxed and filling with blood. (Compare SYSTOLE and see also BLOOD PRESSURE)

diastolic Relating to the DIASTOLE.

diathermy The use of high-frequency electricity to produce heat either in PHYSIOTHERAPY to treat painful muscles or joints, or in surgical operations to burn away unwanted tissue or to seal off small blood vessels.

diathesis A constitutional susceptibility or predisposition to a particular disease.

Dick test An injection into the skin which, by its reaction, shows the patient's susceptibility to SCARLET FEVER.

dietetics The science of nutrition and of prescribing diets for certain illnesses.

dietician An expert in DIETETICS.

differential diagnosis Judging and selecting possible DIAGNOSES from a patient's SYMPTOMS and SIGNS.

digestion The process by which food is broken down and changed into a form that can be absorbed and used by the body. (See DIGESTIVE TRACT)

digestive tract The digestive tract extends from the mouth and oesophagus to the rectum and anus. Food taken in is broken up by the action of digestive juices in the mouth, the stomach, the duodenum and the small intestine. Nutrients are absorbed into the bloodstream through the vessels of the small intestine. Food waste passes on through the colon to the rectum, to be evacuated at the anus. (see page 74)

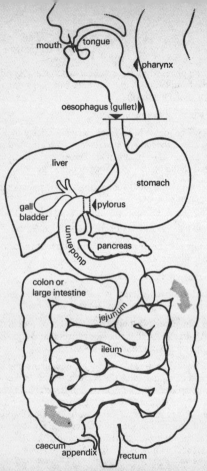

The digestive tract. The liver has been pulled up and back to show the gall bladder on its lower surface.

dilatation and curettage A minor surgical operation in which the opening of the CERVIX of the womb is dilated so that a CURETTE can be passed through and can then gently scrape the lining of the womb. This is done either to provide a sample of the lining for laboratory tests, or to remove undesirable material from within the womb.

diphtheria A serious, acute contagious disease caused by BACILLI and usually affecting the throats of children. It produces a grey-white 'membrane' which can become extensive enough to block the air passage. TOXINS from the bacilli can harm nerves and heart muscle. Treatment includes injections of ANTITOXIN. Once common, diphtheria is now rare because of IMMUNIZATION. (See FEVERS OF CHILDHOOD and also SCHICK TEST)

diplegia Paralysis of similar parts on both sides of the body, for example, both arms or both legs.

diplopia Double vision.

dipsomania see **alcoholism**

disc see **intervertebral disc**

discrete Made up of separate parts; for example, a discrete rash is one consisting of individual spots which do not run together in one area.

disinfectant A chemical used to kill BACTERIA. The term is generally applied to those substances used on objects rather than on people. (See ANTISEPTIC)

dislocation The displacement of a bone from its correct position in a JOINT.

disseminated sclerosis see **multiple sclerosis**

distal Relatively further from the centre of the body. (Compare PROXIMAL)

diuresis Increased production of urine.

diuretic A drug which stimulates and increases the production of urine.

diurnal Occurring during the daytime or period of natural light.

diverticulitis Inflammation of one or more of the pouches present in the colon in DIVERTICULOSIS.

diverticulosis A condition in which small pouches or diverticula form in the COLON and bulge out from weakened points in its walls.

diverticulum (plural, *diverticula)* A small pouch or sac formed in the wall of a hollow organ. See DIVERTICULOSIS.

D.L.E. An abbreviation for disseminated LUPUS ERYTHEMATOSUS.

DNA An abbreviation for DEOXYRIBONUCLEIC ACID.

dorsal 1 Relating to the back. **2** Towards the back of the body. (Compare VENTRAL)

dorsiflexion The bending backwards of joints. In the case of the ankle or wrist it indicates bending the front of the foot or the back of the hand upwards.

dorsum The back or posterior surface of part of the body; for example, the dorsum of the hand compared with the palm.

double-blind In trials of drugs a technique where (until the end of the test) neither the patients nor those who adminster the drugs know which patients have been given an active drug and which an inert substitute.

douche A stream of water or fluid used to flush out or wash a body cavity, for example, a vaginal douche.

Down's syndrome or **mongolism** A congenital condition due to a complex CHROMOSOME abnormality in the CELLS of the patient. The head and face are broad and flat, the eyes slant, the mouth is small and the tongue may protrude, and the hands are stubby. Mental powers are below normal and speech may be poor. The degree to which these features are present can vary considerably.

drachm An old measure of liquid (equals 60 minims) or of weight (equals 60 grains).

dracunculus see **Guinea worm**

drainage In surgery the use of a small rubber tube, temporarily in position, leading from the part operated on to the outside to allow the escape of pus or other fluids.

dressing A protective covering on a wound.

drip A method of introducing fluid into the body, such as nutrients into the stomach or blood into a vein, through a tube with the flow controlled to a drop-by-drop rate.

dropsy An excessive accumulation of fluid in a body cavity or beneath the skin.

d.t. or **d.t.'s** An abbreviation for DELIRIUM TREMENS.

d.t. per vacc. An abbreviation for a combined VACCINE against diphtheria, tetanus and pertussis (whooping cough).

duct A tube leading from a GLAND which carries away its secretions.

ductless glands

ductless glands see **endocrine glands**

ductus arteriosus In the FOETUS, a short blood vessel connecting the two main arteries from the heart – the pulmonary artery which circulates blood through the lungs and the aorta which distributes blood to the rest of the body. It enables blood to bypass the lungs, which do not function before birth. After birth the ductus arteriosus closes and the lungs receive their full circulation. (See PATENT DUCTUS ARTERIOSUS)

Dumdum fever see **kala-azar**

dumping syndrome SYMPTOMS of nausea, faintness, sweating, flushing and occasionally diarrhoea which sometimes occur suddenly after a meal in a patient who has had a PARTIAL GASTRECTOMY.

duodenum The first part of the intestine situated between the stomach and the jejunum. (See DIGESTIVE TRACT)

Dupuytren's contracture A thickening of some of the fibrous tissue in the palm, which pulls on the TENDONS of one or more fingers, flexing them so that they cannot be straightened.

dura mater The outer of the three MENINGES which cover the brain and SPINAL CORD.

d.v.t. An abbreviation for DEEP VEIN THROMBOSIS.

dys- A prefix meaning 'bad', 'faulty', 'difficult' or 'painful'.

dysarthria Difficulty of speech due to lesion in the nervous system or in the muscles concerned.

dyscrasia An abnormal or disturbed condition; a disorder of a body system.

dysdiadochokinesis Inefficient or deranged DIADOCHOKINESIS, associated with disturbance of some parts of the nervous system.

dysentery Infection of the large intestine accompanied by pain and diarrhoea.

dysfunction Abnormal or disordered functioning of an organ.

dysgraphia Inability to write properly due to a disturbance of the nervous system or to the muscles concerned.

dyskinesia Impaired power of voluntary movement.

dyslexia Impaired ability to read and write words correctly; word blindness. This is generally a congenital condition resulting from a brain lesion.

dysmenorrhoea Painful menstrual periods.

dyspareunia Painful or difficult sexual intercourse.

dyspepsia Indigestion pains or discomfort.

dysphagia Difficulty or pain in swallowing.

dysphasia Speech difficulty with impared ability to coordinate and place words in their right order.

dysphonia Impairment of voice.

dyspnoea 1 Difficulty or pain in breathing. **2** Marked shortness of breath.

dystrophy Disorder of an organ or part of the body due to faulty nutrition.

dysuria Difficulty or pain in passing urine.

E **ear** (see opposite)

ecchymosis Extravasation of blood under the skin; a bruise.

eccrine Relating to the sweat glands of the skin.

ECG An abbreviation for ELECTROCARDIOGRAPH.

Echinococcus A kind of TAPEWORM which infests animals like sheep and dogs. It is occasionally transmitted to man and can form CYSTS in different parts of the body, such as the liver or the lungs.

echocardiogram ECHOGRAPHY of the HEART.

echoencephalography ECHOGRAPHY of the BRAIN.

echography The passage of ultrasonic sound waves into the body. The nature of their echoes, which vary with the differing densities of the individual tissues they meet, is recorded electrically to give a picture of the position of or changes in the organs.

echo viruses A group of viruses which can cause serious infections like MENINGITIS and ENCEPHALITIS.

eclampsia Convulsions due to severe TOXAEMIA OF PREGNANCY.

ECT An abbreviation for ELECTRO-CONVULSIVE THERAPY.

–ectomy A suffix meaning 'surgical excision or removal'.

ectopic In an abnormal or displaced position.

ectopic beat A contraction of the heart which is not stimulated through the heart's normal muscle and nerve PACEMAKER mechanism. The occasional ectopic beat can happen in a quite healthy person.

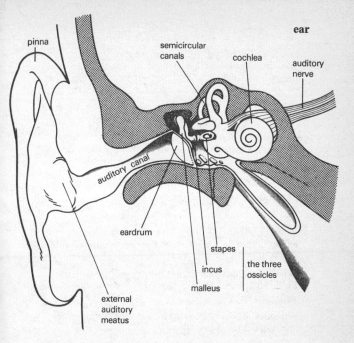

ear

pinna

semicircular canals

cochlea

auditory nerve

auditory canal

eardrum

stapes

incus

malleus

the three ossicles

external auditory meatus

The outer ear. *This includes the pinna and the auditory canal leading to the eardrum. Sound travels down the canal to vibrate the eardrum.* The middle ear. *This contains the three ossicles which transmit the vibrations from eardrum to the base of the cochlea.* The inner ear. *Within the spiral, curved cochlea a fluid transmits the vibrations to nerve endings which carry sound impulses to the brain. The three semicircular canals, each in a different plane, are not concerned with sound but register position and movement of the head.*

ectopic pregnancy Pregnancy in which the fertilized OVUM does not reach the uterus but develops elsewhere – generally in one of the FALLOPIAN TUBES. This can lead to rupture of the tube and the need for an immediate operation.

ectropion The outward turning of the edge of an eyelid.

eczema Inflammation of the skin. There is no definite distinction between it and DERMATITIS, but the term eczema is generally used to cover more CHRONIC forms.

EEG An abbreviation for ELECTRO-ENCEPHALOGRAPH.

effleurage In MASSAGE a light stroking.

effort syndrome see **Da Costa's syndrome**

effusion Outpouring of fluid into a body cavity, for example into the chest or into a joint space, as a result of INFLAMMATION.

ego In psychology that part of the personality which is consciously in touch with the outside world. (See also ID and SUPEREGO)

ejaculation In sexual activity the forceful discharge of SEMEN from the penis.

ejaculatio praecox Orgasm and ejaculation by the male too early in sexual intercourse.

elastic tissue CONNECTIVE TISSUE containing within it a large number of elastic fibres. One of the places where it is found is the wall of arteries.

electrocardiograph An apparatus which records and measures the small, varying, electrical impulses which occur in heart muscle at each beat. By means of leads attached to the patient's limbs and chest, the rhythm, action and state of health of different parts of the heart can be assessed. The record itself is known as an electrocardiogram.

electro-convulsive therapy or **electroplexy** The treatment of some mental disorders by the use of electrically induced fits. This is done by giving the patient a small electric shock to the scalp under carefully controlled conditions.

electro-encephalograph An apparatus which records and measures the small, varying, electrical impulses which occur in the brain. By means of leads attached to the patient's scalp many features of the activity and health of different parts of the brain can be assessed. The record itself is called an electro-encephalogram.

electrolysis The use of electricity to destroy unwanted tissue, for example, HAIR FOLLICLES in cases of HIRSUTISM.

electromyography A method of studying and recording the nerve impulses to muscles and the response of the muscles to them. The record is called an electromyogram.

electroplexy see **electro-convulsive therapy**

elephantiasis Thickening and swelling of the skin and of the tissues beneath due to blockage of the LYMPHATIC vessels in the area. This is most commonly found in the lower limbs in the tropical disease FILARIASIS.

elixir A pleasantly flavoured and sweetened liquid containing a medicine.

embolism The sudden blocking of an ARTERY by an EMBOLUS. (See also PULMONARY EMBOLISM)

embolus

embolus Matter carried in the bloodstream until it blocks an ARTERY. It can be a clot, or air bubble or a particle of fat. The effect depends on the size of the artery, the nature of the tissue it supplies, and whether that tissue has an alternative supply from other arteries. (See also PULMONARY EMBOLISM)

embrocation A LINIMENT.

embryo The developing baby in the womb from the inception of pregnancy until the beginning of the third month. (Compare FOETUS)

emesis Vomiting.

emetic A drug which induces vomiting.

EMG An abbreviation for ELECTROMYOGRAPHY.

emmetropia The correct focusing on the retina of the rays of light entering the eye.

emollient Cream, ointment or liquid used to soothe and soften the skin.

emphysema Abnormal presence or accumulation of air in organs or tissues. (See also SURGICAL EMPHYSEMA and PULMONARY EMPHYSEMA)

empyema A collection of PUS within a natural body cavity. The term is generally used with reference to an ABSCESS between the two layers of the PLEURA.

emulsion A liquid in which fat or oils are held in suspension as a great number of minute globules. This facilitates digestion and absorption in the intestines.

enamel The thin, hard outer layer of the CROWN of the TEETH.

enanthem A rash on a MUCOUS MEMBRANE. (Compare EXANTHEM)

encapsulated Enclosed within a sheet of tissue.

encephalitis Inflammation of the brain.

encephalitis lethargica A form of ENCEPHALITIS which occurred in epidemics but now is rare. It sometimes left permanent mental and physical changes including mental lassitude and certain features of PARKINSON'S DISEASE. It was popularly called 'sleepy sickness', as distinguished from 'sleeping sickness'.

encephal(o)- A prefix meaning 'relating to the brain.'

encephalography An X-ray examination of the BRAIN. The VENTRICLES can be outlined by introducing air or other gas into them before the X-ray is taken.

encysted Enclosed in a CYST or capsule.

endarteritis Inflammation of the inner lining of an ARTERY.

endemic Always present among a certain people or in a certain region, as a disease. (Compare EPIDEMIC and PANDEMIC)

endo- A prefix meaning 'inside' or 'internal'.

endocarditis Inflammation of the endocardium, the lining of the chambers and valves of the heart.

endocrine glands These are glands which secrete HORMONES. The major ones are the pituitary, pineal, thyroid, parathyroid, adrenals, pancreas, testes and ovaries.

endocrinology The study of ENDOCRINE GLANDS and their diseases.

endogenous (Of a condition) due to causes which have arisen within the body itself. (Compare EXOGENOUS)

endometriosis A condition in which TISSUE similar to that of the ENDOMETRIUM is found in sites other than the womb, for example in the ovary, in the abdominal organs or in the skin. This tissue will undergo the same monthly cyclical changes of swelling and bleeding as the ENDOMETRIUM and so cause regular symptoms of pain and swelling.

endometritis Inflammation of the ENDOMETRIUM.

endometrium The lining of the UTERUS.

endorphins The name given to types of OPIATES which appear to be produced by the nervous system of the body and to play a part in controlling pain.

endoscope Any instrument designed to be passed into a body cavity to be examined by a doctor. Many of these specially shaped tubes are fitted with lights and lenses.

endothelium The layer of CELLS which line many body cavities such as the blood and lymph vessels and the heart.

endotoxin A TOXIN which is contained within the substance of BACTERIA. Its damaging effect is limited to the area occupied by the bacteria. (Compare EXOTOXIN)

enema Liquid injected into the RECTUM and the lower part of the COLON to carry medication, to clean the bowel or to help DIAGNOSIS.

engagement The normal state at the end of pregnancy or the beginning of labour when the baby in the womb has settled low, so that its head fits within the upper part of the mother's PELVIS.

E.N.T. An abbreviation for ear, nose and throat.

entamoeba One of several forms of AMOEBA which can live parasitically in the intestines. Some are harmless; others can cause disease.

enter(o)- A prefix meaning 'relating to the INTESTINE'.

enteral or **enteric** Relating to the small INTESTINE.

enteric-coated Describes tablets or capsules covered with a preparation which prevents the absorption of the drug until it has passed the stomach and reached the intestine.

enteric fever A term covering TYPHOID FEVER and PARATYPHOID FEVER.

enteritis Inflammation of the INTESTINE.

enterostomy Surgical construction of an artificial opening between the INTESTINE and the abdominal wall. (Compare COLOSTOMY)

entropion The inward turning of the edge of an eyelid.

enuresis The involuntary passing of urine. In older children bed wetting at night or 'nocturnal enuresis' is only rarely due to a physical disorder. Generally speaking emotional factors are involved, and treatment is therefore psychologically directed.

enzymes Any of the complex proteins produced by some living CELLS to activate many of the chemical changes essential to life within the body.

eosinophil One form of LEUCOCYTE.

eosinophilia The presence in the body of an abnormally large number of EOSINOPHILS. This can occur in some ALLERGIC conditions and in infestation with some PARASITES.

epi-

epi- A prefix meaning 'above' or 'over'.

epicanthus A thin vertical fold of skin at the inner CANTHUS of the eye, normally found in Mongolian people.

epicondyle A prominence on a bone generally near a joint and a site for the attachment of a muscle tendon.

epidemic An outbreak of an infectious disease affecting many people in one region at the same time. (Compare ENDEMIC and PANDEMIC)

epidemic pleurodynia Another name for BORNHOLM DISEASE.

epidemiology The study of the incidence, distribution and spread of diseases.

epidermis The outer layer of the skin. It has one layer of actively growing cells. Outside this are the dead, hard, dry cells which form the surface of the body and which are constantly being shed and replaced from the living layer.

epididymis A long thin coiled tube attached to the back of the TESTIS from which it receives and stores SPERMATOZOA.

epididymitis Inflammation of the EPIDIDYMIS.

epididymo-orchitis Inflammation of the EPIDIDYMIS and TESTIS.

epidural Relating to the space immediately outside the DURA MATER.

epigastrium The upper part of the abdomen.

epiglottis A flap of membrane-covered cartilage lying over the opening of the LARYNX, at the beginning of the TRACHEA (windpipe). When food is swallowed the epiglottis moves down to cover the larynx and prevent food from entering the trachea.

epilepsy A disorder of the brain marked by recurring attacks of temporarily impaired consciousness, often with convulsions and complete loss of consciousness.

In the 'grand mal' form the patient suddenly and silently falls down without warning, although some may experience an AURA and others may utter a single cry. After a brief interval of silent rigidity the patient experiences jerky movements of face, arms and legs for up to thirty seconds. He then passes into relaxed unconsciousness for a variable time before recovering.

'Focal' or 'Jacksonian' epilepsy is a form in which the jerking begins in one part of the body, for example, the hand, and then spreads to other parts, often with no loss of consciousness.

The 'petit mal' form is much simpler, and loss of consciousness lasts only a few seconds.

epiphora Overflowing of the normal tear fluid secretion of the eye as a result of blockage of the LACRIMAL duct.

epiphysis The extremity at either end of a long bone. It begins its development separately from the shaft, to which it is joined by cartilage. After childhood the cartilage is changed to bone, and the shaft and the two epiphyses then become one bone. (Compare DIAPHYSIS)

epiploic Relating to the OMENTUM.

episiotomy A planned incision into the PERINEUM made at the time of DELIVERY in order to widen the outlet of the birth passage. This may be done to ease the birth of the baby and to forestall irregular tearing of the perineum which would require more complicated stitching and a longer healing process than the episiotomy.

epispadias A malformation of the URETHRA in the male, so that it opens somewhere on the front of the penis and not at its tip. Its roof may be wholly or partly lacking. A similar condition may exist in the female, the urethra opening above the CLITORIS. (Compare HYPOSPADIAS)

epistaxis Bleeding from the nose.

epithelioma A TUMOUR arising from the EPITHELIUM.

epithelium The layer of cells providing a covering or lining for body surfaces, such as the skin, or for cavities such as the blood vessels.

epulis A TUMOUR of the gums.

erectile tissue Tissue which when stimulated can become rigid or erect, for example in the NIPPLE, CLITORIS or PENIS.

erogenous Arousing erotic or sexual feelings. Erogenous zones are those parts of the body which produce these feelings when they are stimulated.

erosion The 'wearing away' of a TISSUE; a shallow ULCER.

eruction Belching

eruption 1 A rash. **2** The breaking out and appearance of developing teeth.

erythema Redness in an area of skin.

erythema ab igne A mottled rash of skin due to exposure to heat, as on the legs of people who repeatedly sit close to a fire.

erythema multiforme A skin disease with scattered small areas of redness.

erythema nodosum An ACUTE skin condition with raised red tender lumps. This usually shows on the legs as an ALLERGIC reaction to some infection.

erythroblastosis foetalis Severe HAEMOLYTIC ANAEMIA which develops in the newborn baby as a result of RHESUS FACTOR incompatibility. With modern safeguards and techniques the condition is now not only rare and preventable but also, if it occurs, treatable.

erythrocyte The red blood cell: its function is the carrying of oxygen round the body by means of the HAEMOGLOBIN it contains.

erythrocyte sedimentation rate A laboratory test which measures the speed with which the erythrocytes settle in a column of blood placed in a thin glass tube. A speed higher than normal suggests the activity of certain diseases.

erythropenia An abnormally low number of ERYTHROCYTES.

eschar A slough or scab.

E.S.R. An abbreviation for ERYTHROCYTE SEDIMENTATION RATE.

essential A term used by doctors to describe an abnormal condition which has no obvious cause. (See also IDIOPATHIC)

ethical Relating to drugs whose manufacturers make them available only through a doctor's prescription.

eu- A prefix meaning 'good', 'normal' or 'satisfactory'.

eugenics The science dealing with the GENETIC improvement of the human race.

euphoria An unusually heightened or abnormal sense of elation.

Eustachian canal A narrow canal connecting the back of the throat with the air space in the middle ear. (See EAR)

euthanasia A quiet, painless death. Advocated by some for patients suffering from distressing and fatal diseases.

exacerbation Worsening of a condition.

exanthem A rash on the skin in an infectious fever such as chicken pox or measles. (Compare ENANTHEM)

exanthem subitum Another term for ROSEOLA INFANTUM.

exhibitionism A sexual deviation characterized by a desire to shock people of the opposite sex by exposing the genitals.

exo- A prefix meaning 'outside' or 'external'.

exocrine gland see **gland**

exogenous (Of a condition) due to causes which have arisen outside the body. (Compare ENDOGENOUS)

exomphalos Congenital abnormality of a gap or weakness of the abdominal wall in the region of the navel.

exophthalmic goitre see **thyrotoxicosis**

exophthalmos A condition in which the eyeballs protrude; found with some disorders of the THYROID GLAND.

exotosis A BENIGN growth of bone projecting from the surface of normal bone.

exotoxin A TOXIN excreted by BACTERIA which can have damaging effect on areas of the body other than that occupied by the bacteria. (Compare ENDOTOXIN)

expectorant Medicine designed to assist the coughing up of SPUTUM.

extension The straightening of a JOINT. The opposite of FLEXION, it does not necessarily involve achieving only a straight line between the two parts on either side of the joint. Extending the knee will straighten the leg, but full extension of the wrist joint will draw the hand right back.

extensor A muscle which straightens a JOINT. (Compare FLEXOR)

extra- A prefix meaning 'beyond', 'outside' or 'additional'.

extrasystole A single beat of the heart additional to its normal rhythm and similar to an ECTOPIC BEAT.

extravasation The escape of fluids such as blood, SERUM or LYMPH from vessels into body tissues.

extrinsic factor The name originally used for Vitamin B_{12} in its role of preventing PERNICIOUS ANAEMIA.

extrovert A personality type with interests and activities directed outwards towards exterior events and other people. (Compare INTROVERT)

exudate Fluid which has seeped through the walls of blood vessels into body tissues, generally as a result of INFLAMMATION.

eye (see opposite)

F **facial nerve** The seventh CRANIAL NERVE, it supplies the muscles which control facial expression. It is the nerve involved in BELL'S PALSY.

facial paralysis see **Bell's palsy**

facies The appearance of the patient's face as an indication to DIAGNOSIS.

faeces The waste matter in the colon, which in normal circumstances is eventually expelled through the anus. (See DIGESTIVE TRACT)

Fahrenheit A measurement of degree of temperature shown as °F. It depends on a scale of equal degrees between 32°F for the melting point of ice and 212°F for the boiling point of water. The normal body temperature of a human being is given as 98.6°F, but can range slightly above or below this.

Fallopian tubes The tubes that lead, one from each ovary, to the UTERUS. They convey the ovum from the ovary. (See REPRODUCTIVE SYSTEM, FEMALE)

Fallot's tetralogy A congenital heart malformation consisting of a narrowing of the artery leading to the lung and direct communication between the two VENTRICLES as a result of defect in the wall separating them. This produces extra strain on the right ventricle, which becomes enlarged, and a shift in the position of the AORTA. The child is blue and easily made breathless. (See HEART)

familial Relating to disorders or to bodily or mental characteristics which tend to be found in members of the same family.

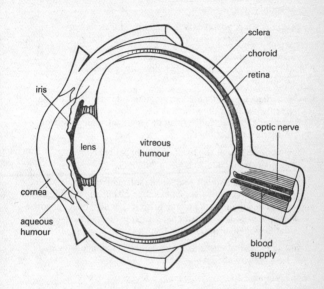

The structure of the eye

farmer's lung An acute asthma-like ALLERGIC reaction to the inhalation of SPORES from some FUNGI. It may occur seasonally in agricultural workers inhaling dust from mouldy hay or grain.

fascia A sheet of FIBROUS TISSUE around muscles or covering other organs.

fasciculation Small, spontaneous contractions of muscles. These may be visible as rippling movements of the overlying skin.

fatty degeneration Excessive accumulation of fat in the TISSUES of an organ which consequently becomes less efficient. It may follow any CHRONIC difficulty in the nutrition of that organ.

fauces The area at the back of the throat between the mouth and the PHARYNX.

favism Severe sudden ANAEMIA resulting from the destruction of ERYTHROCYTES after eating a type of bean, fava, or inhaling its pollen. It is rare, being found in some people who lack an enzyme which protects against the damaging chemical in the bean.

favus A type of TINEA infection of the scalp, producing large yellow crusts.

febrile Relating to, or having, a fever.

fellatio In sexual activity, oral stimulation of the penis.

femoral Relating to the thigh or to the FEMUR.

femoral hernia HERNIA of a loop of the intestine causing a bulge under the skin near the groin. It is near the site of, and may appear similar to, an INGUINAL HERNIA.

femur The thigh bone. (See SKELETON)

fenestration A surgical operation to relieve deafness from OTOSCLEROSIS by making an artificial opening in the LABYRINTH of the ear.

fertilization The union of the SPERMATOZOON and the OVUM; the point at which conception occurs.

fetishism An abnormal mental attitude in which erotic excitement is obtained from an object, such as an article of clothing or from a nonsexual part of the body, such as the foot.

fever Body TEMPERATURE raised above the normal range. It is generally due to infection, though some brain injuries or conditions like HEAT STROKE can cause a rise in temperature.

fevers of childhood (see pages 98–99)

fibreoptics Examination of the interior of hollow organs by using bundles of very thin and flexible fibres which allow light to travel along them.

fibrescope The apparatus used in FIBREOPTICS.

fibrillation Rapid twitching contractions of muscle fibres. (See also AURICULAR FIBRILLATION and VENTRICULAR FIBRILLATION)

fibrin An insoluble PROTEIN derived from the soluble fibrinogen in the blood and forming the basis of COAGULATION.

fibrinogen A chemical in solution in the blood and the precursor of FIBRIN in the process of COAGULATION.

fevers of childhood

Name (common and medical)	Incubation period (days)	Chief features	Approximate isolation period (days)
chickenpox varicella	14–21	Generally mild. Crops of pink spots turning to small blisters – mainly on the trunk and upper thighs.	14
diphtheria	2–4	Severe feverish illness and sore throat with prostration. A 'membrane' may form in the throat interfering with breathing.	Variable. May be for some weeks.
German measles rubella	14–21	Slight fever and sore throat. Rash of many small pink spots, appearing first on face and neck and spreading. Enlarged glands in the neck.	4–7
measles morbilli	10–14	Fever, running nose, watering eyes and cough. Rash of large pink spots beginning	Until 4 days after the rash has cleared.

Name (common and medical)	Incubation period (days)	Chief features	Approximate isolation period (days)
		behind the ears and spreading.	
mumps epidemic parotitis	14–28	Fever, painful swelling of the salivary glands in the face and neck.	Until 5 days after the swellings have subsided.
polio-myelitis	7–14	Headache, sore throat, weakness. In severe forms there is some paralysis.	Variable
scarlet fever scarlatina	1–5	Marked sore throat. Fever. Bright scarlet rash over body. Skin sometimes peels.	Variable
whooping cough pertussis	7–14	Cough begins mildly and gradually worsens to coughing spasms followed by a sharp inspiration (whoop).	Variable

fibroblasts

fibroblasts Cells which develop into various types of CONNECTIVE TISSUE and which form scars in wounds.

fibrocystic disease A hereditary disease characterized by the defective functioning of many glands, including those of the BRONCHI, of sweat and of digestion. The ducts of the PANCREAS become obstructed. The lungs may be blocked with MUCUS and easily infected.

fibroid A fibrous tumour. The term is generally used for the FIBROMYOMA of the UTERUS. It is BENIGN but may give trouble because of its sheer size and by causing bleeding from the lining of the UTERUS.

fibroma A BENIGN tumour of FIBROUS TISSUE.

fibromyoma see **fibroid**

fibrosis The formation of tough, fibrous tissue such as scar tissue.

fibrositis Inflammation of FIBROUS TISSUE, especially of the sheaths of muscles. The term covers a vague set of symptoms including muscular pains and stiffness.

fibrous tissue TISSUE composed of firm fibres and sometimes many elastic fibres, found in many parts of the body filling spaces and covering or connecting different organs.

fibula A bone in the lower leg. (See SKELETON)

filariasis A tropical disease with infestation by thread-like worms, caught through the bite of a mosquito or other insect, which introduces larvae into the patient. The adult worms in the body come to lie in the vessels of the LYMPHATIC SYSTEM and in due course may block these causing ELEPHANTIASIS.

finger-nose test A test for accurate co-ordination of movements related to certain parts of the nervous system. The patient is asked to close his eyes, extend his arm and then touch his nose with the INDEX FINGER.

first aid Emergency help for the injured or sick before medical attention, which can be considered as 'second aid', is available. It aims to preserve life, to prevent the condition from becoming worse and to make circumstances as favourable as possible for recovery.

fissure A crack or split in a MUCOUS MEMBRANE or in the skin.

fistula An abnormal connecting passage between the cavities of two hollow organs, or between the hollow organ and the skin.

fistula-in-ano A FISTULA between the RECTUM and the skin near the ANUS.

flaccid Weak, soft, lax.

flagellum (plural, *flagella*) A minute thread- or whip-like process on MICRO-ORGANISMS, whose movement it helps.

flat foot A flattening of the natural arches of the foot.

flatulence Excessive gas in the stomach and intestines, causing discomfort. Generally gas in the stomach is air that has been unconsciously swallowed and gas in the intestines comes from the digestive breakdown of food.

flatus Gas or 'wind' passed through the back passage.

flexion The bending of a JOINT. (Compare EXTENSION)

flexor A muscle which bends a JOINT. (Compare EXTENSOR)

flexure

flexure 1 A bend or curve, as of an organ. **2** A natural skin fold.

flora In bacteriology a term used to describe the bacteria normally present in a particular part of the body.

fluke A small parasitic worm.

fluoroscopy X-ray examination which enables the image to be seen direct on a fluorescent screen.

flutter A very fast, abnormal but regular, beat of the chambers of the heart.

foetus The developing baby in the womb from the beginning of the third month of pregnancy until birth. (Compare EMBRYO)

follicle A small cavity, sac or gland in the body. (See GRAAFIAN FOLLICLE, HAIR FOLLICLE)

follicle-stimulating hormone A hormone produced by the PITUITARY GLAND which influences the activity of the OVARIES.

folliculitis Inflammation of follicles, generally HAIR FOLLICLES.

follow-up A planned medical check on a patient some time after the end of treatment.

fontanelles These are normal, soft membranous gaps where the separate bones of the newborn baby's skull have not yet united. The largest at the front and top, the anterior fontanelle, closes as the bones unite fully by the age of eighteen months. This point is called the bregma.

foramen A term applied to any of various normal openings or passages in the body.

forceps A two-bladed surgical instrument for handling tissues or dressings. Obstetric forceps are large with curved ends, which are placed around the baby's head to help delivery in the final stages of a delayed childbirth.

forensic Relating to legal matters. Forensic medicine deals with the application of medicine to the law, such as the investigation of accidental or criminal injuries.

foreskin The loose fold of skin which covers the tip of the PENIS.

formication Itching of skin as if it were covered with crawling insects.

fortification figures Patterns of zig-zag coloured lights sometimes experienced as the AURA to a MIGRAINE attack.

fracture A break in a bone.

fracture–dislocation A fracture near a joint accompanied by dislocation of the joint.

fragilitas ossium Another term for OSTEOGENESIS IMPERFECTA.

framboesia see **yaws**

frigidity In a woman the absence of normal sexual feelings or the ability ever to achieve orgasm.

fringe medicine A term used to describe various unorthodox and not completely accepted, but often successful, methods of treatment such as ACUPUNCTURE, OSTEOPATHY or HERBALISM.

Fröhlich's syndrome A condition of obesity and a reduction in genital development due to a malfunctioning of the PITUITARY GLAND.

frontal bone The bone forming the front and upper part of the skull. (See SKELETON)

frostbite Damage to the skin caused by its exposure to severe cold.

frozen section A technique for freezing a piece of tissue from a BIOPSY, allowing it to be quickly cut sufficiently thin for immediate microscopic examination.

frozen shoulder A painful stiffness and limited movement of the shoulder due to inflammation of the membranes enclosing the shoulder joint.

F.S.H. An abbreviation for FOLLICLE-STIMULATING HORMONE.

fugue Abnormal behaviour and actions by a patient, who will not remember them later. They may be due to mental or physical causes.

fulminating Occurring and developing very fast and severely, as a disease.

functional A term used loosely to describe: **1** An abnormal SIGN or SYMPTOM with no detrimental effect, as, for example, an unusual heart sound compatible with complete health. **2** Abnormal working of part of the body without demonstrable physical cause. This then implies a psychological factor.

fundus The base of a hollow organ, such as the EYE or the UTERUS, or the part furthest from its opening.

fungicide A preparation used to destroy FUNGI.

fungus An extremely simple type of plant life whose CELLS generally form a mesh of branching threads. Fungi vary from mushrooms to the microscopic forms which cause TINEA Some, like yeast, exist as separate cells.

funnel chest A congenital deformity in which the breastbone is depressed.

furuncle A boil or skin abscess which has developed from the base of a HAIR FOLLICLE or a SEBACEOUS GLAND. The pus is contained under pressure, which is painful. Attempts to squeeze the pus out are likely to spread it with dangerous results. (See also CARBUNCLE)

furunculosis An outbreak of boils.

fusion The surgical uniting of bones at a JOINT. The immobilizing of the joint in this way is used to relieve severe chronic inflammatory pain.

gait Manner of walking.

G

galactosaemia A rare CONGENITAL condition in which the body cannot perform the normal conversion of GALACTOSE to GLUCOSE.

galactose A simple form of sugar.

gall bladder A sac under the liver in which BILE from the liver is stored before being passed into the DUODENUM. (See DIGESTIVE TRACT)

gallop rhythm On AUSCULTATION, the effect of a third HEART SOUND, giving a rhythm suggestive of the noise of a horse galloping.

gall stone see **calculus**

gamete A male or female CELL for sexual reproduction; a SPERMATOZOON or an OVUM.

gamma globulin A term for any of various PROTEINS found in the blood, which act as ANTIBODIES, protecting against infection.

ganglion 1 A group of nerve cells which act together. **2** A CYSTIC swelling on a tendon or its sheath, usually on the back of the wrist. It is harmless but may become a nuisance because of its size.

gangrene Death of a tissue in one part of the body. It is generally due to a severe reduction of its blood supply.

gargoylism A congenital condition producing dwarf stature, a thickened grotesque face, various abnormalities like deafness and eye lesions, and mental retardation.

gas gangrene Infection by BACTERIA called clostridia which cause complications in injuries. The bacteria thrive on dead or maimed muscle, especially in deep wounds in the absence of air. They also destroy neighbouring healthy tissues, producing gas in the infected area.

gastrectomy Surgical removal of the STOMACH.

gastric Relating to the STOMACH.

gastrin A HORMONE secreted by one part of the STOMACH. It stimulates another part of the stomach to secrete acid and acid juices to digest protein foods.

gastritis Inflammation of the STOMACH.

gastro– A prefix meaning 'relating to the stomach'.

gastro–enteritis Inflammation of both the STOMACH and the INTESTINE.

gastro–enterology The study of the function and diseases of the stomach and intestines.

gastro–enterostomy A surgically made passage between the stomach and the intestine to bypass some part which is diseased, obstructed or has been excised. It is thus a necessary part of a GASTRECTOMY.

gastroscopy Examination of the inside of the stomach by means of a fine tube, with light and optical equipment, which is passed down the OESOPHAGUS.

gastrostomy A surgically made opening into the stomach through the abdominal wall.

gene A minute part of a CHROMOSOME carrying a specific inheritable feature, for example, colour of eyes.

general paralysis of the insane A possible late manifestation of untreated or inadequately treated SYPHILIS many years after the original infection. Extensive damage to the nervous system may lead to emotional instability, mental deterioration, delusions of grandeur, insanity, fits and paralysis.

genetics The study of heredity and inherited characteristics.

genital Relating to reproduction or to the organs of reproduction.

genu The knee.

genu valgum Knock-knee.

genu varum Bow-leg.

geriatrics The medical study of diseases of the elderly and their treatment. (Compare GERONTOLOGY)

German measles A virus infection with a rash, common in children; rubella. (See FEVERS OF CHILDHOOD)

germicide A preparation which destroys BACTERIA.

gerontology The scientific study of the general health and social problems of ageing. (Compare GERIATRICS)

gestation Pregnancy.

giardia PROTOZOAN PARASITES, one form of which may infest the intestines and cause diarrhoea.

gigantism Abnormal enlargement of the whole body due to excess of a HORMONE from the PITUITARY GLAND.

gingiva The gum.

gingivitis Inflammation of the gums.

gland 1 An organ which produces chemical secretion for some specific effect. In exocrine glands the chemicals are led to the site of action through ducts, for example, sweat glands and digestive glands. From ENDOCRINE GLANDS they are carried to more distant sites through the bloodstream. **2** A lymph node of the LYMPHATIC SYSTEM.

glandular fever A virus infection, chiefly of adolescents; infectious mononucleosis. Its features are a sore throat, enlargement of the LYMPH GLANDS, sometimes rashes and, rarely, jaundice. Convalescence may be slow.

glans penis The conical tip of the PENIS.

glaucoma A disease of the eye due to an abnormally high amount of fluid in the eyeball and to high pressure exerted from this on the retina and optic nerve. (See EYE)

glioma A tumour of NEUROGLIA.

globulin A class of PROTEIN found in blood. It includes GAMMA GLOBULIN.

globus hystericus A 'lump in the throat' feeling, related to anxiety or mental tension.

glomerulonephritis see **nephritis**

glomerulus (plural, *glomeruli*) A group of microscopic clusters of blood vessels projecting into the blind end of each minute excretory tubule of the kidney. It is here that the kidney begins its process of filtering chemicals from the blood.

gloss(o)- A prefix meaning 'relating to the tongue'.

glossitis Inflammation of the tongue.

glossopharyngeal nerve The ninth CRANIAL NERVE, it is concerned with the muscles of swallowing and the sense of taste.

glottis In the LARYNX the two vocal cords and the space between them.

glucose A form of sugar and the chief one found in the body. Other forms of sugar taken in food are digested and transformed into glucose. Glucose is used in the body to provide energy.

glue ear A condition in which the middle ear cavity is filled with sticky fluid after repeated attacks of infection treated with ANTIBIOTICS.

gluteal Relating to the buttocks.

gluten A protein found in wheat and other cereals. (See COELIAC DISEASE)

glycaemia The normal presence of GLUCOSE in the blood. (See also HYPOGLYCAEMIA and HYPERGLYCAEMIA)

glycogen Carbohydrate stored in the liver. It is made from GLUCOSE and acts as reserve energy, being broken down to glucose again when needed.

glycosuria The presence of sugar in the urine.

gm An abbreviation for gram.

goitre A swelling of the THYROID GLAND in the neck.

gonad A male or female sex gland: the TESTIS or OVARY.

gonadotropins HORMONES which act on the GONADS. They are formed by the PITUITARY GLAND, but some are also produced by the CHORION during pregnancy.

gonococcus The BACTERIUM which causes GONORRHOEA.

gonorrhoea A VENEREAL DISEASE caused by the bacterium GONOCOCCUS. Within two to ten days after infection the first symptoms – painful and frequent urination and discharge from the URETHRA or VAGINA – may appear. In untreated cases the infection may spread to the TESTICLES or to the womb and FALLOPIAN TUBES. Later damage in untreated cases may include special forms of ARTHRITIS, CONJUNCTIVITIS and ENDOCARDITIS.

gout An illness due to faulty chemical processes in the body, which allow the deposition of uric acid crystals in the tissues, especially at the joints, and particularly the joint at the base of the big toe, which become very painfully inflamed.

G.P.I. An abbreviation for GENERAL PARALYSIS OF THE INSANE.

gr. An abbreviation for grain.

Graafian follicle The small FOLLICLE which forms monthly in an OVARY of a woman of childbearing age and within which an OVUM develops.

grafting The transplanting of a healthy tissue to replace a diseased or damaged one. In an 'autograft' the tissue is taken from the patient's own body. The 'homograft' or 'allograft' uses tissue from another human being and the 'heterograft' tissue from another species.

grain An old weight equal to about 0.065 grams.

Gram's stain A purple dye used in laboratories on bacteria
to be examined microscopically. Those which retain the
blue dye are 'Gram positive'. The others are 'Gram
negative'. This is a helpful preliminary classification of
BACTERIA into two groups.

grand mal see **epilepsy**

granulation tissue In wounds, freshly formed soft tissue,
which precedes scar formation and full healing.

granuloma (plural, *granulomata*) A mass of excessive
GRANULATION TISSUE resulting from a CHRONIC
inflammatory condition.

granuloma inguinale A venereal disease of tropical areas,
characterized by ulcers, with GRANULOMATA on the
genitals.

Grave's disease see **thyrotoxicosis**

gravid Pregnant.

gravida A pregnant woman.

greenstick fracture A crack in a bone which does not go
right across it but may cause it to bend. It occurs chiefly
in children.

grey matter The parts of the brain and spinal cord which
are grey in colour because they contain mainly nerve
tissue without the white MYELIN sheaths which cover the
nerve fibres in those parts called the white matter.

group therapy In psychiatry the treatment of a group of
patients meeting together under the guidance of one
doctor.

Guinea worm or **dracunculus** A tropical parasitic worm. From infested drinking water it reaches the intestine and then migrates within the body to a position under the skin.

gumboil An infectious swelling on a gum, which is generally associated with an abscess at the root of a decayed tooth.

gumma A soft rubbery deposit which can cause a swelling in any part of the body in the tertiary stage of SYPHILIS.

gyn(o)-, gynae- Prefixes meaning 'relating to women'.

gynaecology That branch of medicine and surgery dealing with the diseases of women.

gynaecomastia Enlargement of the breast in males.

gyrus One of the normal convolutions or folds on the surface of the brain.

H **haem(o)-, haemato-** Prefixes meaning 'relating to blood'.

haemangioma see **angioma**

haemarthrosis Extravasation of blood into a joint cavity.

haematemesis Vomiting of blood.

haematocoele Effusion of blood into a body cavity.

haematocolpos Accumulation of blood in the VAGINA. (See IMPERFORATE HYMEN)

haematology The study of blood and its diseases.

haematoma A swelling due to a localized collection of blood (generally clotted) from ruptured blood vessels. A bruise is a haematoma under the skin.

haematuria Blood in the urine.

haemochromatosis A hereditary disease of men in which iron pigment is deposited in many parts of the body including the skin, which darkens, and the PANCREAS, which may cause DIABETES.

haemodialysis The use of DIALYSIS for the purification of a patient's blood by the KIDNEY MACHINE in certain cases of poisoning or kidney failure.

haemoglobin An iron-containing pigment in the ERYTHROCYTES (red blood cells) giving the blood its colour. Oxygen from air in the lungs combines with the pigment to form oxyhaemoglobin. In this way the oxygen is carried by the blood to all parts of the body for the nutrition of TISSUES.

haemoglobinaemia A condition characterized by an excessive amount of HAEMOGLOBIN in the blood.

haemoglobinuria The abnormal presence of HAEMOGLOBIN in the urine.

haemolysis The breakdown of ERYTHROCYTES, with the liberation of their HAEMOGLOBIN into the blood PLASMA. A certain degree of haemolysis is normally always taking place, the cells being replaced by the formation of new ones.

haemolytic anaemia Anaemia due to an abnormal degree of HAEMOLYSIS.

haemolytic disease of the newborn see **erythroblastosis foetalis**

haemophilia An inherited disease marked by defective clotting of blood. The patient tends to bruise easily or to bleed heavily following an injury.

haemoptysis Coughing or spitting up of blood.

haemorrhoids Distended or VARICOSE VEINS under the skin and just within the ANUS; piles.

haemostasis 1 The arrest of bleeding. **2** The control and reduction of blood supply to a part of the body.

haemothorax Blood in the space between the two layers of the PLEURA in the chest.

hair follicles Minute tube-like recesses in the skin from whose bases hairs grow out.

halitosis Offensive odour of the breath. Its causes lie in disturbances and infections of the mouth and teeth, nose and sinuses, throat, lungs, airtubes and stomach.

hallucination Perception by sight, sound or smell of something which is non-existent but which is believed to be real.

hallucinogen A drug likely to produce hallucinations.

hallux The big toe.

hallux valgus A deformity which angles the big toe towards the other toes. It is often due to the wearing of tight shoes.

hamate One of the small CARPAL bones. (See SKELETON)

hammer toe A deformity which arches a toe upwards and backwards. It is often caused by tight footwear.

hamstrings The large muscles at the back of the thigh.

hangnail A small piece of partly detached skin at the base or side of a fingernail.

harelip A congenital defect in which the upper lip has a vertical gap or fissure.

Hashimoto's disease A disease of the THYROID GLAND, with the development of a goitre and inadequate thyroid HORMONE secretion.

hay fever A seasonal ALLERGY caused by sensitivity to airborne pollen and affecting chiefly the eyes and nose.

heart (see page 116)

heart attack A loosely used term to describe ACUTE severe HEART FAILURE or CORONARY THROMBOSIS.

heart block A condition in which the VENTRICLES of the heart fail to respond to and follow the normal beats of the AURICLES, and beat at their own slower rate. (See HEART)

heartburn A burning pain in the upper abdomen and lower chest caused by some digestive disturbance, frequently HIATUS HERNIA. It has nothing to do with the heart.

heart failure Inability of the heart to maintain circulation of blood adequate for the needs of the body.

heart-lung machine An apparatus used during heart surgery which allows the blood to bypass the heart but to continue to take in oxygen and circulate round the rest of the body.

heart massage An emergency first aid measure to try to restore the action of a heart which has suddenly stopped beating. It consists of regularly compressing the heart by pressure on the patient's breastbone. It should be tried only by those properly trained in its use.

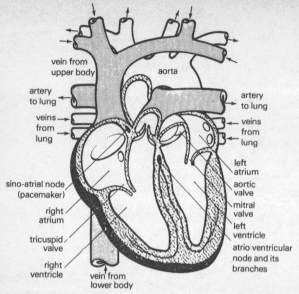

vein from
upper body

aorta

artery
to lung

artery
to lung

veins →
from
lung

← veins
from
lung

sino-atrial node
(pacemaker)

left
atrium

aortic
valve

mitral
valve

right
atrium

left
ventricle

tricuspid
valve

atrio ventricular
node and its
branches

right
ventricle

vein from
lower body

The chambers of the heart *Blood with fresh oxygen comes by veins from the lungs to enter the left atrium and then passes through the mitral valve into the left ventricle. When the ventricle contracts it sends the blood through the aortic valve into the curved beginning of the aorta, the large first artery. Through many arterial divisions it reaches all parts of the body, giving up part of its oxygen to the tissues and then by veins returns to the right atrium. Passing through the tricuspid valve it enters the right ventricle. When this contracts blood is sent through arteries to pick up oxygen again in the lungs.*

The rhythm regulators *(shown very diagrammatically)* are specialized nerve tissues governing the heart beat. The pacemaker, or sino-atrial node, in the wall of the right atrium initiates the beat, spreading impulses through the muscles of the atrial walls. The atrio-ventricular node lower down picks up the impulses and relays them through two conducting branches to the muscles of the ventricle walls.

heart sounds On AUSCULTATION the sounds produced by the heart's action, corresponding to the movement of blood through its chambers and valves and into the first major blood vessels.

heat stroke A dangerous condition marked by an extremely high temperature, failure of the sweating mechanism and collapse after exposure to extreme heat, especially in a moisture-laden atmosphere.

helminth A parasitic worm.

helminthiasis Infestation with HELMINTHS.

hemi– A prefix meaning 'half'.

hemianopia A defect in half the VISUAL FIELD of an eye.

hemiparesis Slight or partial paralysis affecting one side of the body, generally the result of a stroke.

hemiplegia Paralysis of one side of the body, generally as the result of a stroke.

Henoch's purpura A form of PURPURA affecting the inside of the body producing abdominal pain and sometimes blood in the stools.

heparin An ANTICOAGULANT substance produced in the liver and other parts of the body.

hepatic Relating to the LIVER.

hepatic duct The tube through which bile flows from the LIVER. A right and a left duct unite to form the common duct which goes to the GALL BLADDER.

hepatitis Inflammation of the LIVER.

hepatolenticular degeneration see **Wilson's disease**

hepatomegaly Enlargement of the liver.

herbalism A system of treatment based on the theory that in herbs, properly administered, lie the cure for most diseases without danger of side effects.

hereditary (Of a disease) present or latent at birth and inherited through a parent.

hermaphrodite One who has both male and female sexual organs.

hernia The protrusion of an organ, or part of it, through the layers of muscles or other coverings enclosing it; a rupture.

herniorrhaphy Surgical repair of a hernia.

herpes simplex An infection characterized by small blisters which develop around the lips or nose; cold sore. It is due to a virus and may accompany or follow the common cold. It often recurs.

herpes zoster The medical name for SHINGLES.

hetero– A prefix meaning 'other' or 'different'.

heterograft see **grafting**

heterophoria Imperfect balance of the muscles of the eyballs, with failure to keep both eyes pointing precisely. at the object looked at.

heterosexual One who is sexually attracted to persons of the opposite sex.

hiatus hernia A HERNIA of part of the STOMACH through and protruding above the region where the OESOPHAGUS passes through the diaphragm. This allows some of the stomach's acid contents to flow into the oesophagus, where they cause pain. Sometimes food is regurgitated.

hidrosis The production of sweat.

hippus An abnormal and obvious exaggeration of the usually quite slight constant contraction and expansion of the pupil of the eye, irrespective of factors of light and vision. It may be caused by certain nerve troubles.

Hirschprung's disease or **megacolon** A congenital condition in which a part of the COLON becomes grossly distended because of a defect in the nerve supply to the muscles in its wall. The child shows severe constipation and features of INTESTINAL OBSTRUCTION.

hirsutism or **hirsuties** Growth of hair in excessive amounts or on unusual parts of the body, as, for example, on the face of women.

histamine A substance whose presence can cause ALLERGIC reactions. It is found in many animals and plants (e.g., in stings) and it may be released when some TISSUES are damaged. In severe allergies it can cause URTICARIA, tighten air tubes, as in asthma, inflame mucous membranes, as in hay fever, and lower blood pressure, leading to collapse.

histology The study of the microscopic structure of tissues.

Hodgkin's disease or **lymphadenoma** A serious disease characterized by widespread overgrowth of the lymph glands, appearing as swellings at various parts of the body.

homeopathy A system of treatment based on the concept that diseases may be cured by extremely small doses of drugs which, given in ordinary doses to healthy people, could cause the same symptoms as the disease itself.

homo-

homo- A prefix meaning 'same'.

homograft see **grafting**

homosexual One who is sexually attracted to persons of the same sex.

hookworm A parasitic worm which lives attached to the lining of the intestines by minute hooks at its head. The larvae of these worms are found in contaminated water and can penetrate the skin of the feet in order to enter the body.

hordoleum The medical name for STYE.

hormones Chemicals secreted by the ENDOCRINE GLANDS and carried round by the blood, which produce specific actions on various parts of the body distant from the glands themselves.

housemaid's knee Swelling and inflammation of the BURSA in front of the knee. It may develop after frequent kneeling.

Huhner's test Examination of the MUCUS from the CERVIX shortly after intercourse to determine the form and number of SPERMATOZOA. It may be used in the investigation of apparent sterility.

humerus The bone of the upper arm. (See SKELETON)

Huntingdon's chorea A rare hereditary disease of the nervous system which does not show itself until adult life. The patient progressively develops involuntary jerky movements and may in the final stages experience great difficulty with actions like talking, walking or swallowing. It is accompanied by mental disorder. It is unrelated to SYDENHAM'S CHOREA. (See also CHOREA)

Hutchinson's teeth Narrowed INCISOR teeth, with their edge notched. They have been found in congenital syphilis, but may not always be caused by this.

hyaline membrane disease A condition in newborn babies which causes severe breathing difficulties. It is due to the absence of a factor which prevents the minute air sacs of the lungs from collapsing and keeps them dilated. The air tubes of the lungs have a glossy-looking ('hyaline') deposit.

hydatid disease A disease in which cysts containing the larvae of the dog tapeworm form in various parts of the body, including muscles and the liver.

hydatidiform mole A disease of the CHORION. It forms heavy clusters of grape-like VESICLES which fill the uterus. The foetus is destroyed.

hydrocephalus An abnormal accumulation of CEREBROSPINAL FLUID within the brain. It may follow inflammation like MENINGITIS or it may be congenital and cause swelling of the infant's head.

hydrocoele A swelling of the SCROTUM due to fluid forming and collecting in the tissues covering the TESTIS.

hydronephrosis Distension of the kidney due to obstruction of the URETER. (See URINARY TRACT)

hydrophobia see **rabies**

hydrops Another term for DROPSY.

hydrotherapy Use of water in treatment – either externally, as some form of PHYSIOTHERAPY, or internally, as in the drinking of water from mineral springs.

hymen A membrane which partly covers the opening of the VAGINA. It is usually torn during the first experience of sexual intercourse.

hyoid bone A small U-shaped bone at the base of the tongue and above the LARYNX.

hyper- A prefix meaning 'excessive' or 'abnormally increased'.

hyperacusis Abnormally acute hearing or sensitivity to sounds.

hyperaemia An excessive amount of blood in a part of the body; congestion with blood.

hyperaesthesia Abnormally increased nerve sensitivity of an organ. Generally used when referring to the skin's sensitivity to touch, pain or heat.

hypercalcaemia An abnormally high amount of calcium salts in the blood.

hyperchlorhydria An excessive amount of hydrochloric acid in the stomach. The acid plays a part in digestion and in the absorption of iron from foods.

hyperemesis gravidarum Severe vomiting in pregnancy.

hyperglycaemia An abnormally high amount of GLUCOSE in the blood.

hyperhidrosis Excessive sweating.

hyperkeratosis Thickening of the hard outer layer of the skin.

hypermenorrhoea Excessive loss of blood during MENSTRUATION.

hypermetropia Difficulty in focusing on nearby objects; long-sightedness.

hyperpiesis High BLOOD PRESSURE.

hyperpituitarism Excessive secretion of one or more of the HORMONES of the PITUITARY GLAND.

hyperplasia Excessive multiplication and growth of normal cells and TISSUE.

hyperpyrexia An extremely high body temperature.

hypersensitivity Abnormally high sensitivity and body reaction to foreign matter. (See ALLERGY)

hypertension High BLOOD PRESSURE. 'Benign' hypertension is a mild form. 'Malignant hypertension' is more severe and likely to cause complications affecting the heart and blood vessels.

hyperthyroidism Overactivity of the THYROID GLAND.

hypertrophy An abnormal increase in the size of an organ, due to an increase in the size (not the number) of its constituent CELLS.

hyphaema Bleeding within the anterior chamber of the EYE.

hypnosis see **hypnotism**

hypnotic 1 Relating to HYPNOTISM. **2** A drug used to induce sleep.

hypnotism The technique of inducing hypnosis – a trance-like or semi-conscious state with a very high response to suggestion.

hypo-

hypo- A prefix meaning 'beneath' or 'deficient in'.

hypoaesthesia Abnormally lowered nerve sensitivity of an organ. Generally used when referring to the skin's sensitivity to touch, pain or heat.

hypocalcaemia An abnormally low amount of calcium salts in the blood.

hypochlorhydria Deficiency of hydrochloric acid in the stomach. (Compare ACHLORHYDRIA)

hypochondria Excessive concern and worry about one's health and about trivial or imagined ailments.

hypochondrium The outer side of the upper part of the abdomen, lying under the lower ribs.

hypochromic anaemia ANAEMIA characterized by an abnormally low amount of haemoglobin in the ERYTHROCYTES.

hypodermic Under the skin – with specific reference to injections of medicaments under the skin.

hypogammaglobinaemia An abnormally small amount of GAMMA GLOBULIN in the blood.

hypogastrium The lowest part of the middle abdominal region.

hypoglossal nerve The twelfth CRANIAL NERVE, it supplies the muscles of the tongue.

hypoglycaemia An abnormally low amount of GLUCOSE in the blood.

hypomenorrhoea Reduced duration or amount of blood flow in MENSTRUATION.

hypophysis Another name for the PITUITARY GLAND.

hypopituitarism Inadequate secretion of one or more of the HORMONES of the PITUITARY GLAND.

hypoplasia Inadequate or incomplete development of a TISSUE or ORGAN.

hypopyon Pus in the anterior chamber of the EYE.

hypospadias A malformation of the URETHRA in the male, which opens on the underside of the penis and not at its tip. A similar condition may exist in the female, with the urethra opening into the vagina. (Compare EPISPADIAS)

hypostasis Poor circulation of blood in a dependent part of the body.

hypotension Abnormally low BLOOD PRESSURE.

hypothalamus A part of the BRAIN below the third ventricle. Connected by nerve fibres to several other parts of the brain, it is concerned with many functions of the body including emotions, appetite, thirst, temperature, the PITUITARY GLAND and the AUTONOMIC NERVOUS SYSTEM.

hypothenar Relating to the thickened area of the palm between the little finger and the wrist.

hypothermia A very low body temperature, with a slowing down of vital functions, after exposure to cold.

hypothyroidism Abnormally low activity of the THYROID GLAND.

hypoxia An abnormally low level of oxygen supply to the tissues.

hysterectomy Surgical removal of the UTERUS.

hysteria A neurosis arising out of anxiety or frustration in which the patient presents bodily SYMPTOMS as an expression of mental disturbance.

hystero– Relating to the UTERUS.

I **iatrogenic** Describes an illness or abnormality inadvertently produced by the treatment of the original disease.

ichthyosis A hereditary condition of rough, dry, scaly skin.

icterus Jaundice.

icterus gravis neonatorum Another term for ERYTHROBLASTOSIS FOETALIS.

id In psychology the most primitive part of a personality, involving basic drives and instincts. (See also EGO and SUPEREGO)

idiocy Very severe mental deficiency.

idiopathic Describes an abnormal condition which has developed without any obvious cause. (See also ESSENTIAL)

idiosyncrasy An individual's abnormal subsceptibility or reaction to a drug.

I.D.K. An abbreviation for INTERNAL DERANGEMENT OF THE KNEE.

ileitis Inflammation of the ILEUM.

ileostomy Surgical construction of an artificial opening between the ILEUM and the abdominal wall to permit the evacuation of its contents.

ileum The lower part of the small intestine. (See DIGESTIVE TRACT)

ileus Obstruction of the intestine, preventing the passage of its contents.

ilium The haunch bone; one of the bones which forms part of each half of the pelvis. (See SKELETON)

i.m. An abbreviation for INTRAMUSCULAR.

immunity State of resistance to an infection. After recovery from some infectious diseases the patient's system will have reacted by producing ANTIBODIES to the MICRO-ORGANISM concerned. These remain to protect him against further infection from that micro-organism. (See also IMMUNIZATION)

immunization The creation of IMMUNITY to a specific infection. 'Active immunization' consists of administering the appropriate MICRO-ORGANISM in a form so altered or weakened that it will not produce the disease but will still stimulate the development of the appropriate ANTIBODIES. This immunity takes some time to develop and lasts from several months to many years, according to the disease in question. 'Passive immunization' consists of injecting the ready prepared antitoxin. Immunity is then achieved immediately, but lasts only a short time.

immunosuppressive Describes drugs which reduce the body's reaction against foreign matter introduced into it. These are of importance when a surgical TRANSPLAN-TATION from another person is made.

impacted Wedged, jammed or pressed against something.

impacted fracture A fracture in which the broken ends of the bones are firmly wedged into each other.

impacted tooth A tooth which cannot erupt normally through the gums because it is growing out of alignment and jammed against a neighbouring tooth.

imperforate anus An abnormality at birth in which the opening of the ANUS is absent.

imperforate hymen A condition in which the HYMEN is without an aperture and completely closes off the vagina. At the onset of the periods this will cause HAEMATO-COLPOS.

impetigo A CONTAGIOUS infection of the skin due to STAPHYLOCOCCI.

impotence In men inability to achieve or maintain erection of the penis for sexual intercourse.

incarcerated Describes a HERNIA which has become too big to be REDUCIBLE.

incisional hernia A HERNIA through an area of the abdominal wall which has been weakened by an incision in a previous operation.

incisors The front teeth.

incisor teeth see **teeth**

incompatible (Of drugs) unsuited to be administered together because of possible adverse reactions.

incontinence Inability to control bowel or bladder action.

incoordination Failure of the muscles of a part of the body to work with controlled and smooth action. This is generally due to some defect in the nervous system.

incubation The provision of the right conditions for experimental growth in the laboratory of MICRO-ORGANISMS or TISSUE cultures.

incubation period The lapse of time in an infectious disease between the INFECTION of the patient and the appearance of the first SYMPTOMS.

incubator 1 In BACTERIOLOGY an apparatus for holding CULTURES. **2** In maternity units equipment for protecting premature babies. The incubator maintains optimum conditions of temperature and humidity.

incus One of the three small bones which transmit soundwaves within the EAR.

index finger The finger next to the thumb.

indolent (Of a lesion, such as an ulcer or tumour) slowly developing and causing little pain.

induction of labour Artificial means of starting labour when this has been unduly delayed or when it is necessary for the health of the mother or baby.

induration Hardening of a tissue or organ.

infant In medical terms a child up to the age of one year.

infantile paralysis Another name for POLIOMYELITIS.

infant mortality rate In a country or community the annual number of deaths of INFANTS per thousand live births.

infarct or **infarction** Death of a tissue, and ultimately its scarring, through blockage of its blood supply.

infection The penetration of and multiplication in the
body of harmful living organisms like BACTERIA, VIRUSES
and FUNGI. They may enter through a break in the skin
(for example, wounds and stings), with air through the
nose and mouth into the lungs and its tubes (for example,
the common cold and measles), by being swallowed into
the digestive tract (for example, food poisoning), or
through the genital tracts (for example, VENEREAL
DISEASES). Occasionally harmless bacteria, normally
present in one part of the body, such as the bowel, may
spread to another part, for example, the bladder, which
is not resistant to them.

infectious mononucleosis The medical name for
GLANDULAR FEVER.

infertility Inability to conceive or to father children.

infestation The presence of PARASITES on or in the body,
for example, on the hair or skin or in the intestines.

inflammation A defensive reaction of tissues to injury or
infection. The blood vessels in the affected area swell and
allow some of their contents to ooze out, carrying
protective substances, including LEUCOCYTES, to destroy
bacteria or foreign particles. The area develops the
characteristic features of swelling: redness, warmth, pain
and reduced fumction.

influenza An acute viral infection which tends to appear as
epidemics.

infra-red radiation Invisible radiation below the red end
of the spectrum. It is used in PHYSIOTHERAPY for its
heat-producing effect in body tissues.

ingestion Taking a preparation by mouth.

ingrowing toenail A condition in which the free end of a closely cut nail grows into and causes INFLAMMATION in the adjacent skin fold.

inguinal Relating to the groin.

inguinal hernia A HERNIA of a loop of the intestine causing a bulge under the skin near the groin. It is near the site of, and may appear similar to, a FEMORAL HERNIA.

innervation The nerve supply to an organ or structure of the body.

innocent (Of tumours) BENIGN.

inoculation The introduction of MICRO-ORGANISMS or infective material either to a laboratory CULTURE or, as method of IMMUNIZATION, into the body.

insertion The point at which a muscle or its tendon is fixed to the bone which it moves.

insight A psychiatric term to express the extent of a patient's awareness of his mental illness.

insufflation Blowing a gas or powder into a body space.

insulin A HORMONE produced by the PANCREAS to allow the body to use sugar in the blood for energy and tissue building and to regulate the level of that sugar.

integument Skin.

intensive care (In hospital) close and constant supervision and treatment of a patient whose condition may suddenly alter.

inter- A prefix meaning 'between'.

intercostal Relating to the spaces between the ribs.

intercurrent Describes an illness which develops in addition to another already present.

interdigital In the space between adjoining toes or fingers.

intermittent claudication A condition due to narrowed arteries in the leg. Inadequate blood supply causes pain in the muscles after the patient has walked a short distance. Brief rest eases this, but pain and limping or claudication return after walking is resumed.

internal derangement of the knee A condition in which a torn MENISCUS interferes with the function of the knee. Surgical removal of the meniscus may be needed as treatment.

interstitial In the spaces or between the parts of a TISSUE.

intertrigo Chafing and INFLAMMATION of two skin surfaces which are in contact with each other.

intervertebral disc A thick pad of fibrous cartilage between and attached to each VERTEBRA. It has a jelly-like centre. The discs act as buffers and contribute to the movement and stability of the VERTEBRAL COLUMN. The 'slipped disc' is one partly disrupted by a strain on the vertebral column. If it presses against nerves arising from the spinal cord it can cause a disabling pain.

intestinal obstruction A blockage of the intestines which prevents the passage of FAECES.

intestine The part of the DIGESTIVE TRACT which extends from the lower end of the stomach to the anus.

intra– A prefix meaning 'inside' or 'within'.

intracranial Within the skull.

intracutaneous or **intradermal** Within the tissue of the skin.

intramuscular Within the muscle.

intrathecal Within the cover of the spinal cord and into the subarachnoid space and its cerebrospinal fluid. (See MENINGES)

intrauterine device A CONTRACEPTIVE in the form of a small flexible spring, generally made of plastic, inserted within the uterus.

intravenous Within or into a vein.

intravenous pyelogram X-ray examination of the kidneys after the injection into a vein of the arm of a substance which is carried to the kidney by the bloodstream and is opaque to X-rays.

intrinsic factor see **pernicious anaemia**

introvert A type of personality with interests and thoughts directed mainly inwards towards himself or herself. (Compare EXTROVERT)

intubation The insertion of a tube into a cavity or passage of the body.

intussusception Blockage of the intestine caused by part of it being drawn within itself.

in vitro Describes a chemical or bacteriological process undergone in laboratory apparatus, literally 'within glass'.

in vivo Describes a chemical or bacteriological process undergone in the living body.

involution The return of the UTERUS to its normal size after childbirth.

ionizing radiation Radiation of great energy which can produce ions (electrically charged atoms or groups of atoms) in some materials against which it is directed.

ipsilateral On the same side of the body as something already referred to.

iridectomy Surgical excision of a small part of the iris, performed in some treatments of GLAUCOMA.

iridocyclitis Inflammation of the IRIS of the eye and of the structures around it.

iris The coloured ring of the EYE, whose central opening is the pupil.

iritis Inflammation of the IRIS.

irreducible Describes a HERNIA whose protrusion cannot be flattened except by operation.

ischaemia Inadequate blood supply to a part of the body.

ischium One of the two bones forming the lower part of the pelvis. (See SKELETON)

islets of Langerhans A group of cells in the PANCREAS which produce the HORMONE INSULIN.

isolation The segregation of a patient with an infectious disease until the risk of his passing it on has disappeared.

isotope A variant of a chemical element which has the properties of that element. If a RADIOACTIVE isotope can be introduced into the body its presence and distribution can be studied by means of apparatus which registers the radioactivity. This can be used in some cases to diagnose the condition of organs which take up the element.

itis- A suffix meaning 'inflammation'.

i.u.d. An abbreviation for INTRAUTERINE DEVICE.

i.v. Intravenously; by injection into a vein.

i.v.p. An abbreviation for INTRAVENOUS PYELOGRAM.

Jacksonian epilepsy see **epilepsy**

J

jactitation Jerky, uncontrolled movements of the body.

jaundice A yellow discoloration of the skin and of the whites of the eyes caused by excessive quantities of the bile pigment, bilirubin, in the blood.

jejunum Part of the small intestine. (See DIGESTIVE TRACT)

joint The junction of two or more different bones of the body. The bones may be fixed (as in the CRANIUM) or movable (as in the limbs).

jugular Relating to the neck or throat.

Kahn test A blood test for the diagnosis of SYPHILIS.

K

kala-azar A severe tropical infection, one form of LEISHMANIASIS. After an INCUBATION PERIOD of several weeks the symptoms include fever, weakness, marked anaemia, bleeding, and enlargement of the liver and spleen.

keloid An excessive amount of thick hard scar tissue present at a healed wound, cut or burn.

keratin The hard PROTEIN which is a component of hair, nails and other horny tissues, and is also present in the thin outer skin layer.

keratitis Inflammation of the CORNEA.

kerato- A prefix meaning 'relating to the CORNEA' or 'relating to hard or horny tissue'.

kerato-acanthoma A benign skin tumour forming a
round shiny PAPULE with a central depression. It tends to
regress and heal spontaneously.

keratosis A hard or horny growth, for example, a wart.

kernicterus A condition of damage to the brain and the
nervous system following some severe forms of
jaundice.

Kernig's sign A condition characteristic of meningitis:
with the patient lying down and his thigh bent against
the abdomen, any attempt to straighten his knee fails and
causes pain.

ketones Chemicals (including acetone) produced in the
body under certain abnormal conditions, such as severe
diabetes and starvation.

kidney One of the two organs in the body which filter out
waste substances from the blood and maintain the salt
and water balance. (See URINARY TRACT)

kidney machine An apparatus through which a patient's
blood is passed for purification by DIALYSIS. It is used in
certain cases of kidney failure and poisoning.

Kienböck's disease A progressive softening and
degeneration of the lunate bone at the wrist.

kinaesthesia The awareness of the position in space and
movement of the body and limbs.

kleptomania A compulsive desire to steal, even objects of
no value, caused by a mental disturbance.

knee jerk The REFLEX kick which a bent and relaxed leg
gives when tapped sharply just below the kneecap.

koilonychia Thin, concave nails found in some cases of anaemia.

Koplik's spots Very small white spots on a red base found on the gums and on the inside of the cheeks in the early stages of measles.

Korsakov's syndrome An illness with brain deterioration due to various types of poison, including alcohol, and associated with vitamin B deficiency. Its features are loss of memory of recent events, disorientation in time, a tendency to talk about non-existent events, and irritability.

kraurosis vulvae Thinning and dryness of the skin and mucous membranes of the external genitals of women, a condition found mainly in the elderly.

Kveim test A test on the skin to detect the presence of SARCOIDOSIS.

kwashiorkor Severe malnutrition with great protein deficiency. It is common in small children in tropical Africa.

kyphoscoliosis Double curvature of the spine, both backwards and sideways.

kyphosis Backward angulation of the spine; hunchback.

labile Unstable, likely to change.

L

labium (plural, *labia*) A lip or, specifically, the two 'labia majora' and the two 'labia minora', the large and small fleshy folds which form the borders of the VULVA.

labour The process at childbirth of contractions of the uterus by which the baby is born.

labyrinth The inner part of the EAR.

labyrinthitis Inflammation of the LABYRINTH.

laceration An uneven, ragged wound.

lacrimal Relating to glands, ducts, etc. concerned in the secretion of tears.

lacrimal gland A gland in the eye which secretes tear fluid. (See EYE)

lacrimal system That part of the eye which produces, stores and conducts the tear fluid. The LACRIMAL GLAND, tucked above the upper and outer part of the eyeball, normally secretes just enough tear fluid to keep the front of the eye moist. The fluid then drains into the nose through a series of small canals, which start from a minute opening at the edge of each lid near the nose. (See EYE)

lactation The formation of milk in the breasts.

lallation A childish, babbling form of speech.

lamella A very small gelatine disc holding medicament, which is inserted under the eyelid for the treatment of certain conditions.

laminectomy Surgical removal of part of the back of a VERTEBRA to be able to reach the SPINAL CORD.

lancet A small pointed surgical knife with two cutting edges.

lancinating (Of pain) sharp or cutting.

lanugo The very fine hairs on the body of the newborn baby.

laparoscopy The use of an ENDOSCOPE for examining the interior of the abdominal cavity.

laparotomy Surgical incision through the abdominal wall; any operation which opens the ABDOMEN.

large intestine The part of the intestine which runs from the end of the small intestine to the anus. (See DIGESTIVE TRACT)

laryngismus Spasm of the LARYNX.

laryngitis Inflammation of the LARYNX.

laryngoscope An instrument for examining the inside of the LARYNX. It uses an illuminated tube or mirror which is passed to the back of the mouth.

larynx The complex of cartilage and muscles in the neck at the upper end of the TRACHEA which form the 'voice box'. Its prominence in the front of the neck is the Adam's apple. It contains the two vocal cords whose varying tensions and movements create sound as air passes between them.

lassa fever A severe virus infection occurring in West Africa, with high fever, muscle pains, mouth ulcers and prostration.

lateral To the side; away from the mid-line of the body. (Compare MEDIAL)

laughing gas The popular name for nitrous oxide gas, sometimes used as an inhalation for its property of relieving pain.

lavage Washing out or irrigation of a body cavity such as the stomach.

l.e.

l.e. An abbreviation for LUPUS ERYTHEMATOSUS.

legionnaire's disease A BACTERIAL disease resembling PNEUMONIA. Symptoms may include shortness of breath, chest pains, muscle ache and diarrhoea.

leiomyoma A benign tumour of smooth MUSCLE.

Leishmaniasis A group of diseases caused by a microscopic PARASITE (Leishmania) transmitted by the bite of infected sandflies. It includes skin ulcers under various names such as Delhi boil, or Oriental, Baghdad or Tropical sore, and also KALA-AZAR.

lens That part of the EYE which by its alteration of shape focuses the image on to the retina.

lentigo A freckle.

leprosy A CHRONIC bacterial disease of tropical and subtropical areas, with an INCUBATION PERIOD of a year or very much longer. It affects mainly skin and nerves. The skin shows red nodules and later loses colour and thickens. Nerves may thicken and a burning or tingling sensation may be experienced, eventually leading to loss of the sense of touch and sometimes paralysis. As a result deformities may occur in hands and limbs.

leptomeninges The inner two (pia mater and arachnoid) of the three membranes which form the MENINGES taken together.

lesbian A female HOMOSEXUAL.

lesion Any localized injury or disease process.

leuco– A prefix meaning 'white'.

leucocytes These are the white blood cells. They are classified as granulocytes (of three kinds: neutrophils, eosinophils and basophils), lymphocytes and monocytes. The names derive from Greek terms indicating their microscopic appearance and their response to the dyes used for examining them. The cells have varied functions. The granulocytes, for example, provide protection against infection and can move from the bloodstream to tissues to destroy bacterial invaders. The lymphocytes help to form ANTIBODIES.

leucocytosis An increase in the number of LEUCOCYTES in the blood.

leucoderma see **vitiligo**

leuconychia White streaks or spots on the nails.

leucopenia An abnormally low number of LEUCOCYTES in the blood.

leucoplakia The formation of irregular white patches on MUCOUS MEMBRANES. They may be found in the mouth or in the female genital organs.

leucorrhoea Any excessive white discharge from the VAGINA.

leucotomy Surgical severing of some nerve fibres in the front of the brain as treatment for certain severe and otherwise intractable mental illnesses.

leukaemia A MALIGNANT disease involving a vast increase in the numbers of LEUCOCYTES, in immature form, in the bloodstream.

l.g.v. An abbreviation for LYMPHOGRANULOMA VENEREUM.

libido 1 Sexual desire. **2** In PSYCHOANALYSIS the sum total of all instinctive energies and desires; psychic energy.

lichenification

lichenification Thickening and hardening of the skin.

lichen planus A skin disease characterized by scaly or rough blotches which cause itching.

lie (Of the foetus) the way the length of its body lies in relation to that of the mother. In a 'longitudinal' lie the long axis of the foetus is parallel to the long axis of the mother. In a 'transverse lie' it is across it. (See also PRESENTATION)

ligament 1 A tough fibrous band supporting and connecting the bones at a joint. **2** Any band of tissue supporting an organ.

ligature A thread of silk, CATGUT or wire used in surgery to tie and constrict a blood vessel or other structure.

lightening The mother's feeling of reduced abdominal tension when, towards the end of pregnancy, the baby's head becomes engaged in the pelvis and the UTERUS descends a little.

linctus A syrupy medicine, generally one used to relieve a cough.

lingual Relating to the tongue.

liniment A liquid preparation which when rubbed into the skin acts as a COUNTERIRRITANT to relieve pain.

lipaemia An abnormally large amount of LIPIDS in the blood.

lipid One of various fats and fatlike substances, such as cholesterol.

lipoid One of a large number of fat-like substances.

lipoidosis One of a number of rare diseases associated with faulty METABOLISM of LIPOIDS.

lipoma A soft BENIGN tumour of fatty tissue.

lipomatosis A large accumulation of fatty tissue or of many LIPOMAS in one part of the body.

lithiasis The formation of CALCULI in an organ.

lithotomy The surgical removal of a CALCULUS.

lithotomy position A position in which the patient lies on the back with hips and knees flexed, used in some examinations or operations. It is so called, since in the past this position was used for LITHOTOMY operations on the bladder.

lithotrite A surgical instrument for crushing CALCULI in the bladder, after being passed through the URETHRA.

Little's disease A form of congenital CEREBRAL PALSY with spasticity of the limbs.

liver This very large organ, lying under the lower ribs on the right side of the body, has many functions. It secretes BILE for digestion. It performs a great number of chemical tasks essential to life, including the processing of digested material brought to it by the PORTAL VEIN. It breaks down and re-synthesises proteins, neutralizes poisons and stores substances like GLYCOGEN, copper, iron and VITAMINS.

liver flukes FLUKES which can reach the liver and obstruct the BILE DUCT. They can be caught from eating infected vegetables or infected raw fish.

livid Discoloured, bruised.

loa

loa An African threadworm transmitted through the bite of infected flies. It causes severe itching by burrowing under the skin.

lobar pneumonia Infection of the lung confined to one or more of its lobes. (See LUNGS) (Compare BRONCHO-PNEUMONIA)

lobectomy Surgical excision of one of the lobes of a LUNG.

lobotomy Surgical division of nerve tracts in the brain as treatment of some otherwise intractable mental disorders.

local Short for local anaesthetic. (See ANAESTHESIA)

lochia The normal discharge from the VAGINA which takes place for about two weeks after childbirth.

lockjaw see **tetanus**

locomotion The ability to walk or to move from one place to another.

locomotor ataxia A form of ATAXIA, more usually known as TABES DORSALIS.

locum tenens A doctor standing in to do the work of a colleague who is temporarily absent.

loiasis Infestation with LOA.

long sightedness Difficulty in focusing the vision on nearby objects, although distant objects are clearly seen.

lordosis Forward curvature of the spine.

Ludwig's angina INFLAMMATION and ABSCESS formation in the floor of the mouth.

lues An old name for SYPHILIS.

lumbago Pain in the lower part of the back.

lumbar Relating to the loins or the region of the loins.

lumbar puncture The insertion of a hollow needle between two of the lumbar VERTEBRAE into the SPINAL CANAL either to take a sample of the CEREBROSPINAL FLUID or to inject a drug.

lumbo-sacral joint The joint at the base of the spine between the lowest (fifth) lumbar VERTEBRA and the SACRUM. (See SKELETON)

lumen The space or channel within any tubular body, organ or passage.

lungs (see page 146)

lupus erythematosus One of the COLLAGEN DISEASES. Two forms of lupus erythematosus are described. Discoid Lupus Erythematosus presents as a scaly red rash across the nose and, butterfly-shaped, extending over the cheeks. It is made worse by sunlight. Systemic or Disseminated Lupus Erythematosus may also present such a rash, but involves many other parts of the body as well, and may, for example, cause arthritis or defective functioning of the kidneys. Neither has any connection with LUPUS VULGARIS.

lupus vulgaris A form of tuberculosis affecting the skin and generally the face. The condition is rare today.

luxation Dislocation.

lymph see **lymphatic system**

lymphadenitis Inflammation of the LYMPH GLANDS.

lymphadenoma see **Hodgkin's disease**

lungs

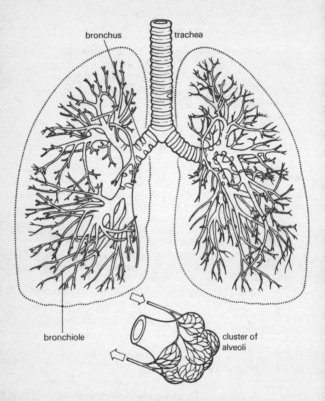

lymphadenopathy Disease of the LYMPH GLANDS.

lymphangiectasis Dilatation of the lymph vessels.

lymphangioma Overgrowth of some tissues of the lymphatic system forming spaces containing lymph fluid.

lymphangitis Inflammation of the lymph vessels. It may show as red streaks in the skin from the area of an infected wound.

lymphatic system A system of thin vessels carrying lymph fluid all over the body. The vessels eventually drain into large veins at the neck. At their connecting points they are set with LYMPH GLANDS or NODES which act as filters for bacteria and foreign particles, and so help prevent the spread of infection. The glands also form LYMPHOCYTES and ANTIBODIES.

lymph glands or **lymph nodes** Masses of lymph tissue set along the LYMPHATIC SYSTEM. They act as formation centres for LYMPHOCYTES and as defence barriers against infection.

lymphocyte One type of LEUCOCYTE or white blood cell.

Movements of the diaphragm and of the chest muscles expand and contract the chest, drawing air in and out of the lungs through the trachea. the trachea divides into two bronchi. Inside its lung each bronchus divides many times into air tubes, leading finally to the alveoli or air sacs. Each minute alveolus is surrounded by capillary blood vessels. Here oxygen is taken into the bloodstream and carbon dioxide is expelled from the bloodstream to be breathed out.

lymphogranuloma venereum A venereal disease found in tropical regions which is due to a VIRUS-like micro-organism. It causes marked swelling of the LYMPH GLANDS in the groin and thickening of the skin in that area.

lymphoma A tumour-like growth of some element of the LYMPHATIC SYSTEM.

lysis 1 Disintegration of a CELL, specifically of ERYTHROCYTES. **2** The gradual abatement of a fever or disease (Compare CRISIS)

M

McBurney's point In a patient with appendicitis the point of maximal tenderness. It is two-thirds of the way down a line between the navel and the front prominence of the hip bone.

macro- A prefix meaning 'large'.

macrocephaly Abnormal largeness of the head.

macule A small discoloured flat spot on the skin. (Compare PAPULE)

Madura foot or **maduromycosis** A tropical fungus infection, generally in the foot, but also affecting other parts of the body and causing swelling and SINUS formation.

malabsorption Deficient absorption of nutrients by the intestines.

malaise A general feeling of being unwell.

malar Relating to the cheek.

malaria A disease caused by four different varieties of a PARASITE called Plasmodium and transmitted by the bite of an infected mosquito. It is found in Africa and Asia, and in Central and South America. The parasites undergo complex changes both in the mosquito and in man. In man they cause attacks at intervals of two or three days or, in the most severe cases, irregularly and more frequently. The attacks consist of a high fever with headache and vomiting, preceded by shivering and followed by heavy sweating and prostration. Complications include anaemia, kidney failure, and brain and lung disturbances.

malignant Describes a relatively severe illness likely to be progressive or recurring. A malignant TUMOUR can harm by.dissemination or invasion within the body.

malingering Deliberate feigning or exaggeration of symptoms of disease.

malleolus The bony projection at each side of the ankle.

mallet finger A finger whose tip is half bent and cannot be straightened, as a result of damage to the tendon which would normally straighten it.

malleus One of the three small bones which transmit soundwaves within the EAR.

malocclusion Imperfect alignment of the teeth in both jaws when the mouth is closed.

malpractice Culpably faulty or unskilled medical or surgical treatment.

Malta fever One form of BRUCELLOSIS.

malunion Defective healing and union of the broken ends of a fractured bone.

mammary Relating to the breast.

mammography X-ray examination of the breast.

mammoplasty Plastic surgery of the breast.

mandible The bone of the lower jaw.

mania A mental condition characterized by over-activity and excitement, often with unjustifiable self-confidence. It can reach a degree of uncontrollable excitement and elation.

manic–depressive One who is subject to alternating states of mania and depression.

manipulation Treatment designed to correct faulty positions of bones and joints by moving or pressing on parts of the body.

Mantoux test A test for recent or past TUBERCULOSIS infection in a patient by noting the reaction of the skin to an INTRACUTANEOUS injection of TUBERCULIN.

manubrium The upper part of the sternum or breastbone.

marasmus Extreme wasting due to malnutrition or MALABSORPTION, especially in children.

march fracture A fracture of one of the METATARSAL bones in the foot, caused by undue exertion like prolonged walking.

Marfan's syndrome A hereditary condition marked by great length of limbs, toes and fingers, heart abnormalities, instability of joints, and disorder of the lenses of the eyes.

marrow A soft red or yellow substance within the inner cavities of bones. Red marrow is concerned with the formation of blood cells.

marsupialization The surgical conversion of a closed cavity of the body into an open pouch by incising it and stitching the cut edges to the edges of the skin wound.

masochism A perversion in which sexual satisfaction is achieved by experiencing pain.

massage Treatment of soft tissues, for example, muscle, by applying friction to or by kneading or stroking part of the body.

mastectomy Surgical excision of a breast.

mastication Chewing.

mastitis Inflammation of the breast.

mastoidectomy Excision of the air cells of the MASTOID PROCESS in order to drain away pus.

mastoiditis Inflammation of the air cells within the MASTOID PROCESS.

mastoid process The bony swelling just behind the lobe of the ear. It contains a honeycomb of air cells which connect, through a small opening, with the inside of the ear.

maxilla The bone of the upper jaw.

maxillary sinus see **antrum**

measles A virus infection, with a rash, commonly occurring in epidemics in children. The medical name is morbilli. (See FEVERS OF CHILDHOOD)

meatus An opening or passage to an organ.

Meckel's diverticulum A small appendix-like protrusion from the ILEUM, present in about one person in fifty.

meconium

meconium The dark green, semifluid contents of the baby's bowels at birth, which are passed soon after. It contains chiefly mucus and bile.

medial Towards the mid-line of the body. (Compare LATERAL)

mediastinum The space within the chest between the two lungs. Its contents include the heart, OESOPHAGUS, THYMUS GLAND and the lower part of the TRACHEA.

medulla oblongata The lowest part of the brain stem, continuing as the uppermost part of the SPINAL CORD.

megacolon see **Hirschprung's disease**

megalomania Delusions of grandeur; an unshakeable conviction of one's greatness.

megrim An old name for MIGRAINE.

Meibomian cyst Blockage and swelling of a MEIBOMIAN GLAND.

Meibomian glands SEBACEOUS GLANDS situated at the edge of the eyelid.

melaena Stools which appear tarry black, discoloured by bleeding in some part of the digestive tract.

melancholia A severe state of DEPRESSION.

melanin A dark pigment which colours skin, hair and eyes.

melanoma A TUMOUR of pigment-producing CELLS. It can be BENIGN or it may become MALIGNANT.

membrane see **mucous membrane**

menarche The age at which the menstrual periods first appear.

Ménière's syndrome A condition associated with disturbance of the inner EAR and reduced hearing. It produces sudden attacks of severe VERTIGO and TINNITUS, often with nausea and vomiting. The attacks last from a few minutes to several hours and appear at irregular intervals of days or months.

meninges A threefold layer which covers the brain and SPINAL CORD. The outer layer, the tough and fibrous DURA MATER, is attached to the inside surface of the skull and (more loosely) of the vertebrae. The middle layer is the ARACHNOID. The inner layer, the thin and delicate PIA MATER, is attached to the surface of the brain and spinal cord. Between the ARACHNOID and the PIA MATER is the subarachnoid space containing the CEREBROSPINAL FLUID.

meningism Symptoms like those of MENINGITIS without in fact involvement of the meninges.

meningitis Inflammation of the MENINGES. Fever, severe headache, stiffness of the neck and back, and difficulty in bending the head forwards are some features of meningitis.

meningococcal meningitis MENINGITIS caused by infection from bacteria called meningococci. It is the commonest form of MENINGITIS and, because of a characteristic rash which may appear, is also known as 'spotted fever'.

meningocoele Protrusion of the MENINGES through a gap in a faultily developed VERTEBRA. (See also SPINA BIFIDA)

meniscectomy Surgical removal of a MENISCUS.

meniscus or **semilunar cartilage** One of two crescent-shaped pads of fibrous cartilage between the bones of the knee joint.

menopause The 'change of life' in women; the time when MENSTRUATION and reproductive ability come to an end.

menorrhagia Abnormally heavy bleeding during menstruation.

menses The monthly periods.

menstruation Periodic bleeding (usually monthly and lasting about four days) from the vagina of sexually mature women who are not pregnant. It comes from the natural breaking up of the lining of the womb. Any very irregular bleeding or bleeding after the MENOPAUSE needs medical advice.

meralgia paraesthetica Pain and abnormal sensation in the outer part of the thigh, due to disturbance of the nerve supplying this area.

mesentery A large fold of PERITONEUM around and supporting the intestines.

meta- A prefix meaning **1** 'after'. **2** 'changing', 'transforming'.

metabolism The sum of all the chemical and energy changes in the body responsible for maintenance of growth and repair, for the conversion of complex substances into simpler ones, and for their reconstruction into body materials.

metacarpal Relating to the area of the hand between the fingers and the wrist and to the bones within it.

metastasis The spread of a disease from one part of the body to a quite different part. The term is generally used in connection with malignant tumours.

metatarsal Relating to the area of the foot between the toes and the ankles and to the bones within it.

meteorism Distension of the abdomen resulting from gas in the intestines.

metritis Inflammation of the womb.

metropathia Any disorder or disease of the womb.

metropathia haemorragica Abnormal thickening of the lining of the womb, associated with heavy and irregular periods.

mg and **mgm** Abbreviations for MILLIGRAM.

microbe see **micro-organism**

microcephaly Abnormal smallness of the head, generally associated with abnormal brain development and mental deficiency.

micro-organism Any living organism too small to be seen without a microscope, for example BACTERIA, VIRUSES, PROTOZOA and some FUNGI.

micturition Urination; passing urine from the bladder.

midstream specimen or **midstream urine** A urine specimen specially collected for laboratory testing. The patient interrupts the passing of urine to resume and to collect in a sterile bottle some of that which is subsequently passed. This ensures that the specimen is free from accidental contamination.

migraine Attacks of headache occurring irregularly and lasting some hours. They are often preceded by an AURA of flashing or zig-zag sensation of light (FORTIFICATION FIGURES). Generally they affect one side of the head only and are frequently accompanied by PHOTOPHOBIA, nausea and vomiting.

milaria

milaria see **prickly heat**

miliary tuberculosis TUBERCULOSIS which is scattered widely through the body as small points of infection.

milligram A weight equal to one thousandth of a gram.

millilitre A liquid measure equal to one thousandth of a litre.

Milroy's disease A hereditary condition characterized by swelling of the legs. Its cause is uncertain.

minim An old measure of fluid amounting to approximately one drop or one-sixtieth of a DRACHM.

miotic A drug which produces miosis, i.e. contraction of the PUPIL of the eye.

miscarriage A popular name for ABORTION.

mitral stenosis Narrowing of the opening of the MITRAL VALVE.

mitral valve A valve in the HEART lying between the left atrium and the left ventricle.

mittelschmerz Abdominal pain in women at the time of OVULATION, mid-way between two menstrual periods.

ml An abbreviation for MILLILITRE.

molar teeth see **teeth**

mole A raised, pigmented spot on the skin.

molluscum contagiosum A virus infection of the skin which develops small nodular swellings.

molluscum fibrosum see **neurofibromatosis**

mongolism A former name for DOWN'S SYNDROME.

Monilia or **Candida** A yeast-like fungus which can infect skin or mucous membranes. In the vagina it produces an irritant discharge. In the mouth it causes THRUSH.

mono– A prefix meaning 'one' or 'single'.

monocular Relating to one eye only.

monocyte A type of LEUCOCYTE.

monocytosis or **mononucleosis** An abnormally high number of MONOCYTES in the blood. (See LEUCOCYTES and INFECTIOUS MONONUCLEOSIS)

monoplegia Paralysis of a single part of the body.

mons pubis or **mons veneris** In women, the rounded swelling of skin overlying the bones above the VULVA.

morbid (Of a part of the body) diseased.

morbilli The medical name for MEASLES.

moribund Nearing death.

motor nerve see **nerve**

motor neurone disease Any disease of nerves controlling muscles, with loss of power in those muscles.

M.S. An abbreviation for MULTIPLE SCLEROSIS.

mucopus MUCUS and PUS mixed.

mucosa A mucous membrane.

mucous membrane A delicate membrane lining cavities of the body, such as the air tubes, digestive tract and the nose, and secreting MUCUS.

mucus A viscid fluid secreted by mucous membranes which keeps them moist, as in the nose. IN INFLAMMATION or ALLERGIC reaction of the membranes the secretion may become thick and excessive.

multi- A prefix meaning 'many'.

multigravida A pregnant woman who has been pregnant before.

multipara A woman who has borne several children.

multiple myeloma A MALIGNANT tumour in the bone marrow which can cause marked bone damage.

multiple sclerosis A slowly progressive disease in which the insulating MYELIN sheath protecting the nerves degenerates and the affected nerves develop patchy SCLEROSIS at scattered points in the body. The onset is insidious and the results vary according to which nerves are damaged and lose their function. Symptoms, which may include dizziness, numbness, visual troubles, and weak or stiff limbs, often have phases of REMISSION and RELAPSE.

mumps A virus infection affecting the SALIVARY GLANDS. (See FEVERS OF CHILDHOOD)

Münchausen syndrome The habitual seeking of hospital admission by giving a plausible but a false history of illness and by simulating symptoms.

murmur A sound heard on AUSCULTATION, in particular an abnormal heart sound.

muscle An ORGAN which by its contraction produces movement of part of the body. There are three types. Striated or striped muscle is under voluntary control and can move a limb. Smooth or plain muscle is under unconscious control, an example being that which activates the intestines. Cardiac muscle is that which makes the heart beat rhythmically.

muscular dystrophy A hereditary disease causing progressive weakness and wasting of muscles.

my(o)- A prefix meaning 'relating to muscle'.

myalgia Pain in the muscles.

myasthenia Weakness of muscle.

myasthenia gravis An illness characterized by progressive weakening of the muscles in the body. It is due to a defect in the transmission of nerve impulses into the muscles.

mycology The study of FUNGI.

mycosis Any disease caused by FUNGUS.

mydriasis Dilation of the PUPIL of the eye.

myel(o)- A prefix meaning **1** Relating to the marrow. **2** Relating to the SPINAL CORD.

myelin A white, fatty substance which forms the protective sheath round nerve fibres.

myelitis 1 Inflammation of the MARROW. **2** Inflammation of the SPINAL CORD.

myelocoele Protrusion of the SPINAL CORD through a defect in a VERTEBRA.

myelography An X-ray examination to determine the outline of the spinal cord, after injecting a fluid opaque to X-rays into the CEREBROSPINAL FLUID filling the subarachnoid space. (See MENINGES)

myeloma A tumour of the marrow.

myocarditis Inflammation of the heart muscle.

myocardium The heart muscle.

myoma A tumour of muscle tissue.

myopathy Any disease of the muscle.

myopia Short-sightedness.

myosarcoma A MALIGNANT tumour of muscle.

myositis Inflammation of muscle.

myotonia An abnormal spasm or contraction of muscles.

myringitis Inflammation of the ear drum.

myringoplasty Plastic surgery on the ear drum.

myringotomy Surgical incision of the ear drum to allow the escape of pus which has formed behind it.

myxoedema A condition due to prolonged reduction of THYROID GLAND activity. The skin becomes thick and dry, the hair thins, the patient becomes slow and overweight and very sensitive to cold.

N

naevus A birthmark on the skin caused either by abnormal pigmentation or by a mass of tiny blood vessels.

narcoanalysis The use of NARCOTICS as an aid in psychoanalysis.

narcolepsy A condition in which the patient, otherwise normal, has sudden uncontrollable attacks of sleepiness.

narcosis Sleepiness or stupor caused by a drug.

narcotic A drug which produces NARCOSIS.

nares The nostrils.

nasal Relating to the nose.

naso– A prefix meaning 'relating to the nose'.

nasal bone One of two small bones forming the bridge of the nose. (See SKELETON)

nasolacrimal duct The passage which drains tear fluid from the eye into the nose. (See LACRIMAL SYSTEM)

nasopharynx The part of the PHARYNX behind and above the soft PALATE. It connects with the back of the nose.

naturopathy A system of treatment using natural diets and physical methods and avoiding drugs.

nausea A sensation of sickness and of being likely to vomit.

navicular Another term for SCAPHOID bone (in either foot or hand.)

nebulizer An apparatus for administering a drug as a fine spray, for example, to be sniffed up the nose or inhaled through the mouth.

necro– A prefix meaning 'relating to death'.

necropsy see **autopsy**

necrosis The death of a tissue or organ.

neonatal Relating to the first four weeks after birth.

neonate A newborn infant.

neoplasm A 'new growth' – the medical name for TUMOUR.

nephrectomy Surgical removal of a kidney.

nephritis Inflammation of the kidney, also known as glomerulonephritis, that is, inflammation of the filtering glomeruli (see KIDNEY). ACUTE nephritis appears to be an allergic reaction to a STREPTOCOCCAL infection elsewhere in the body, as the throat, from which the patient suffered about two weeks previously. Features are fever, blood and PROTEIN in the urine, and OEDEMA. Most patients recover fully but a few may develop the chronic form.

   CHRONIC nephritis can be insidious, slow developing and long-lasting. In many cases the SYMPTOMS are slight but in others it may turn into the state known as NEPHROSIS.

nephro– A prefix meaning 'relating to the kidneys'.

nephroblastoma A cancerous tumour of the kidney which develops in infancy.

nephrolithiasis Stones in the kidney.

nephron One of the microscopic filtering units of the kidney.

nephrosis or **nephrotic syndrome** A group of conditions in which malfunction of the kidneys from one of several causes, including NEPHRITIS, produces severe OEDEMA and the passage of much PROTEIN into the urine, with consequent loss of protein from the blood.

nephrostomy Surgical incision into the kidney, for example, to remove stones.

nerve A bundle of fibres conveying impulses of feeling or of motion between parts of the body and the brain or spinal cord. Motor nerves carry only impulses to activate muscles; sensory nerves carry only those of sensation. Most nerves carry both types.

neuralgia Pain along the course of a nerve.

neurasthenia An ill-defined condition of weakness and lassitude, accompanied by slight depression.

neuritis Inflammation of a nerve.

neuro- A prefix meaning 'relating to nerves'.

neurofibromatosis A hereditary condition marked by the formation of fibrous swellings on the nerves (neurofibroma) and pigmented blotches on the skin.

neurogenic 1 Forming or stimulating nerve tissue. **2** Arising from the nervous system.

neurogenic bladder Loss of function and control of the bladder due to damage to its nerve supply.

neuroglia CONNECTIVE TISSUE in the brain and spinal cord.

neuroleptic see **tranquillizer**

neurology The study of the nervous system and its diseases.

neuroma A tumour of the nerve cells.

neuropathy Any abnormal condition in the nervous system. The term is generally used of those parts which are beyond the brain.

neurosis Any sustained abnormal mental condition in which the sufferer has altered behaviour or beliefs without losing his sense of reality. He is aware that he is mentally disturbed. (Compare PSYCHOSIS)

neurosyphilis SYPHILIS which affects the nervous system.

neutropenia An abnormally low number of NEUTROPHILS in the blood.

neutrophil A type of LEUCOCYTE.

night blindness Inability to see in a dim light. It may be associated with a deficiency of Vitamin A. (See VITAMINS)

nipple The pigmented projection at the centre of the breast. It holds the openings of the ducts through which the baby sucks milk.

nit The egg of a louse.

nocte A prescription indication meaning 'at night'.

nocturia Excessive urination at night.

node 1 Any small mass of tissue. **2** See LYMPH GLANDS. **3** Any of several small areas of special tissues in the heart which control the rate of heart beat. (See HEART)

noma Another term for CANCRUM ORIS.

normo- A prefix meaning 'normal' or 'usual'.

normoblast An early stage in the formation of an ERYTHROCYTE or red blood cell.

normocytosis Normal condition of the ERYTHROCYTE contents of the blood.

nosocomial Relating to a or originating in a hospital.

nosology The classification of diseases.

notifiable disease A disease whose occurrence must be notified to the health authorities so that preventative action against its spread may be taken, or so that statistical information may be collected.

n.p. A prescription indication: the name of the drug to be written on the label of the container – the initials of the Latin words 'nomen proprium'.

nucleus A spherical body within a CELL, controlling its essential living factors and determining its characteristics and inherited features.

nucleus pulposus The soft centre of the INTERVERTEBRAL DISC. Its displacement may be the causative factor in a 'slipped disc'.

nullipara A woman who has never borne a child.

nymphomania Excessive sexual desire in a female.

nystagmus A rapid involuntary movement of the eyes from side to side or up and down. It may occur in certain nerve disorders.

obstetrics The branch of medicine dealing with the care of women during pregnancy, childbirth and the weeks immediately after.

obstruction see **intestinal obstruction**

occipital bone The bone at the back and base of the skull. (See SKELETON)

occiput The back of the head.

occlusion The fit between the teeth of the upper and lower jaws when both jaws are closed.

occult blood Blood present in FAECES or other matter in such small amounts that it is detectable only by special tests.

occupational disease A disease caused by adverse or unhealthy working conditions, as, for example, exposure to fumes or the action on the skin of chemicals.

O

occupational therapy Use of some form of planned and supervised work as part of the treatment of a patient.

oculentum Ointment for application to the eye.

oculomotor nerve The third CRANIAL NERVE, it supplies the muscles controlling the movements of the eyeball and eyelid.

o.d. A prescription indication meaning 'every day' – the initials of the Latin words 'omni die'.

odont- A prefix meaning 'relating to teeth'.

odontology Dentistry.

oedema An abnormal accumulation of fluid in the tissues, causing puffiness.

Oedipus complex Sexual feelings of a son towards his mother.

oesophagus The tube connecting the throat with the stomach; the gullet. (See DIGESTIVE TRACT)

oestrogen One of the female HORMONES produced by the OVARIES, it is responsible for the sexual characteristics of the female body and also plays a part in controlling the menstrual cycle.

olecranon The bony point of the elbow, at the upper end of the ulna. (See SKELETON)

olfactory Relating to the sense of smell.

olfactory nerve The first CRANIAL NERVE, it transmits the sense of smell.

oligaemia Insufficient volume of blood in the body.

oligo- A prefix meaning 'few' or 'little'.

oligospermia Deficiency of SPERMATOZOA in the SEMEN.

oliguria Decreased production of urine.

o.m. A prescription indication meaning 'every morning' – the initials of the Latin words 'omni mane'.

-oma A suffix meaning 'tumour'.

omentum A large loose fold of PERITONEUM which hangs from the stomach and COLON and lies over the intestines.

omphalo- A prefix meaning 'relating to the navel'.

omphalocoele A congenital defect of the abdominal wall at the UMBILICUS, with protrusion of some of the intestine.

o.n. A prescription indication meaning 'every night' – the initials of the Latin words 'omni nocte'.

onco- A prefix meaning 'relating to TUMOURS'.

oncology The study and treatment of TUMOURS.

onychia Inflammation under a nail.

onychogryphosis Marked overgrowth, thickening and deformity of a nail.

oopho- A prefix meaning 'relating to the OVARIES'.

oophorectomy Surgical removal of an OVARY.

oophoritis Inflammation of an OVARY.

ophthalmia Severe inflammation of the eye with CONJUNCTIVITIS.

ophthalmia neonatorum Acute CONJUNCTIVITIS in a newborn baby caused by contamination at birth.

ophthalmology The study and treatment of eye conditions.

ophthalmoplegia Paralysis of the eye muscles.

ophthalmoscope An instrument for examining the inside of the eye.

opiate A drug containing opium or a similar preparation; a NARCOTIC.

opisthotonos A muscular spasm which arches the body strongly backwards. It is due to severe irritation of the nervous system.

optic disc The area in the RETINA where the OPTIC NERVE leaves the eye and enters the base of the brain. It shows as a small pink or white circle.

optic nerve The nerve carrying visual sensation from the eye to the brain.

oral 1 Relating to the mouth. **2** (Of drugs) administered by mouth or to be swallowed. (Compare PARENTERAL)

orbit The eye socket.

orchi– A prefix meaning 'relating to the TESTIS'.

orchidectomy Surgical removal of a TESTIS.

orchidopexy Surgical correction and fixation in the SCROTUM of an UNDESCENDED TESTICLE.

orchitis Inflammation of the TESTIS.

organ A distinct part of the body with its own definite functions, such as the brain, kidneys, lungs, etc.

organism Any individual living plant or animal form, irrespective of size and complexity.

orgasm The climax of emotional and physical excitement in sexual activity.

oriental sore see **Leishmaniasis**

ornithosis An infectious disease of birds transmittable to humans and causing a pneumonia-type illness. (See also PSITTACOSIS)

ortho- A prefix meaning 'straight' or 'correct'.

orthodontics Dentistry concerned with the correct position and regularity of teeth.

orthopaedics The treatment of abnormalities and deformities occurring in bones and joints, including fractures.

orthoptics Treatment by exercise of defects of the eye muscles.

os calcis see **calcaneus**

–osis A suffix meaning 'a diseased condition'.

ossicle 1 A very small bone. **2** One of the three small linked bones which transmit sound waves in the middle ear. (See EAR)

osteitis Inflammation of a bone.

osteitis deformans A slowly progressive condition marked by softening of the bone, followed by thickening and deformity. The spine, the bones of the leg and the skull are especially affected.

osteoarthritis A chronic disease of the joints, especially the larger weight-bearing ones, with degeneration and partial loss of their smooth CARTILAGE linings.

osteoarthrosis Another name for OSTEOARTHRITIS.

osteochondritis Inflammation of bone and cartilage.

osteochondritis dissecans OSTEOCHONDRITIS at a joint which causes a piece of cartilage and bone to become free and loose in the joint space.

osteoclastoma A bone tumour.

osteogenesis imperfecta A hereditary condition characterized by abnormally brittle bones which are liable to fracture easily.

osteoma A tumour of bone, usually a BENIGN one.

osteomalacia Softening of bone due to insufficiency of minerals in its structure.

osteopathy A system of treatment based on the theory that if it is structurally sound the body itself is capable of curing diseases. The osteopath aims to correct structural defects by bone and joint manipulation and by other methods.

osteophyte A bony outgrowth or excrescence.

osteoporosis Thinning and weakening of bone substance, due to loss of calcium and other minerals. It is more common in the elderly and after prolonged immobilization.

osteosarcoma A MALIGNANT tumour of bone.

–ostomy A suffix meaning 'an artificial opening', used in medicine to indicate a surgically created one, as in COLOSTOMY.

otitis Inflammation of the ear. The words 'externa', 'media' and 'interna' are added for the condition in the outer, middle and inner ear respectively. (See EAR)

otolaryngology The study and treatment of diseases of the ear, nose and throat.

otology The study of the ear.

otosclerosis A thickening and hardening of the structures linking the three OSSICLES of the middle ear, causing deafness.

ovariectomy Surgical removal of an OVARY.

ovary The two ovaries, situated near the UTERUS at the base of the abdominal cavity, are the female sex glands. Their two main functions are to release a mature OVUM (the female reproductive cell) each month and to secrete the female sex HORMONES – OESTROGEN and PROGESTERONE.

oviduct Another term for the FALLOPIAN TUBE.

ovulation The release of an OVUM from the OVARY.

ovum (plural, *ova*) The female reproductive cell.

oxyhaemoglobin see **haemoglobin**

oxytocin A HORMONE secreted by the PITUITARY GLAND. It stimulates contractions in the pregnant UTERUS.

oxyuris see **threadworm**

pacemaker 1 The SINO-AURICULAR NODE of the heart which sends out rhythmic impulses initiating the heart beats.
2 An electronic device worn by a patient, or implanted in his body, to stimulate or regulate the heart beat in certain cases of abnormal heart rhythm.

P

paediatrics The branch of medicine dealing with the diseases and care of children.

Paget's disease 1 Of bone (see OSTEITIS DEFORMANS). **2** Of the nipple: an inflammatory cancerous skin rash around the nipple.

palate The roof of the mouth, also forming the floor of the nose cavity. The front part, containing a plate of bone, is hard.

palliative A treatment which relieves SYMPTOMS but does not aim to cure.

palpebral Relating to the eyelids.

palpitations Awareness of one's own heart beat. This does not necessarily indicate a diseased heart, but sometimes causes unjustified anxiety.

palsy Paralysis.

paludism Malaria.

pancreas A gland in the abdomen behind the stomach possessing a dual function. It secretes digestive juices, which empty into the DUODENUM through a special duct. It also acts as an ENDOCRINE GLAND, secreting INSULIN into the blood as a HORMONE.

pancreatitis Inflammation of the pancreas.

pandemic An EPIDEMIC which is world-wide or covers a very large area. (Compare ENDEMIC)

pannus An overgrowth on the CORNEA consisting of tissue with small blood vessels.

Papanicolaou test A test carried out on cells used for a CERVICAL SMEAR to detect early cancer.

papilla A small projection or elevation above a surface.

papilloedema An oedema swelling at the OPTIC DISC of the eye.

papilloma A benign growth on the skin or MUCOUS MEMBRANE; a wart or POLYP.

papule A small firm raised spot on the skin. (Compare MACULE)

paracentesis The surgical puncturing of a body cavity with a syringe needle to remove fluid, such as pus.

paracusis Any abnormality of hearing.

paraesthesia An abnormal feeling such as 'pins and needles', without any outside cause.

paralysis Loss of power to move muscles in some part of the body.

paralysis agitans An old name for PARKINSON'S DISEASE.

paralytic ileus ILEUS resulting from loss of activity of the muscles of the intestine.

paranoia A mental disorder characterized by firmly held DELUSIONS of persecution or of grandeur and self-importance.

paraphasia A form of APHASIA in which the patient uses wrong words or gets words confused.

paraphimosis Tightness of the retracted FORESKIN of the penis, causing swelling of the GLANS beyond it.

paraplegia Paralysis of the lower part of the body.

parasite A plant or animal which lives on or within the body, from which it obtains its nutriment. Although the term includes bacteria and viruses, it is generally used for animals like worms and insects. (Compare COMMENSAL)

parasympathetic nervous system see **autonomic nervous system**

parathyroid gland One of four ENDOCRINE GLANDS in the neck, whose HORMONE controls the amount of calcium in the blood.

paratyphoid fever A bacterial infection of the intestines very similar to TYPHOID FEVER, but in general less severe. The bacteria are found in both man and animals.

parenchyma The tissues of an organ containing its specific and characteristic cells. (Compare STROMA)

parenteral (Of drugs) not administered by mouth but by some other method, such as injection.

paresis Slight or partial paralysis.

parietal bone One of the two bones forming the upper part and sides of the skull. (See SKELETON)

Parkinson's disease or **Parkinsonism** A slow, progressive degeneration of certain deep brain centres, with gradual and variable development. The features may include, to a varying degree, all or some of the following: stiffness of muscles, poorly coordinated movements, expressionless face, tremor of limbs, twitching of the thumb against the index finger, stooping, and a slow shuffling walk which sometimes swings out of control into a short-stepping run.

paronychia Infection around a nail; a whitlow.

parotid gland The largest of the SALIVARY GLANDS, situated at the cheek below the ear.

parotitis Inflammation of the PAROTID GLAND. 'Epidemic parotitis' is a medical term for MUMPS.

paroxysmal tachycardia An attack of very rapid beating of the heart, which generally starts and ceases suddenly.

partial gastrectomy Surgical removal of part of the stomach.

partial mastectomy Surgical excision of part of a breast.

parturition Childbirth.

passive exercise and movements Those in which a part of the body, for example, a limb, is moved by someone else, such as a physiotherapist, while the patient relaxes. (Compare ACTIVE EXERCISE AND MOVEMENTS)

pasteurization Controlled heating of milk or other fluid to destroy harmful bacteria.

patella The kneecap. (See SKELETON)

patent Open, unobstructed.

patent ductus arteriosus A congenital condition in which the DUCTUS ARTERIOSUS fails to close after birth. Thus a large amount of blood poor in oxygen enters the main circulation without having been enriched by oxygen from the lungs. This is one of the possible causes of a BLUE BABY.

patho- A prefix meaning 'disease'.

pathogen A substance or MICRO-ORGANISM capable of producing disease.

pathology The study of the cause and effects of disease as seen in the changes in TISSUES and ORGANS.

-pathy A suffix meaning 'diseased condition'.

patulous Distended or widely open.

Paul-Bunnell reaction A blood test used to help diagnose GLANDULAR FEVER.

p.c. A prescription indication meaning 'after food' – the initials of the Latin words 'post cibum'.

pectoral Relating to the chest.

pectus excavatum The medical term for FUNNEL CHEST.

pediculosis Infestation with lice.

pediculus A louse.

pellagra A disease caused by deficiency of vitamin B. It produces inflammation in the mouth, anaemia, skin rashes, diarrhoea and sometimes impairment of mental faculties.

Pelligrini Stieda's disease CALCIFICATION of a ligament of the knee which develops as a result of injury.

pelvimetry Measurement of the PELVIS, especially in relation to its internal capacity to let the baby's head pass through during labour.

pelvis The girdle of bones at the base of the abdomen connected to the lower part of the vertebral column.

-penia A suffix meaning 'deficiency'.

penis The male organ of COPULATION. Its channel, the URETHRA, also conveys urine from the bladder.

pepsin An ENZYME in the stomach juices which breaks down PROTEINS.

peptic ulcer An ULCER in the lining of the stomach or DUODENUM.

percussion A diagnostic method which consists of tapping smartly on part of the body, for example, the chest, and judging the underlying condition by the resonance or dullness of the sound produced.

peri- A prefix meaning 'around' or 'near to'.

periarteritis Inflammation of the outer part of an ARTERY and of the surrounding area.

periarteritis nodosa see **polyarteritis nodosa**

pericarditis Inflammation of the pericardium.

pericardium The membranous sac around and enclosing the heart. Its double layer contains a film of fluid which acts as a lubricant during movement.

perinatal Relating to the period (approximately one month) before and after the birth of a child.

perinephric Around the kidney.

perineum Anatomically this is the area between the lower part of the buttocks and the top of the thighs. In practice the word is used to describe the region of skin between the genitals in front and the ANUS behind.

periodontal Relating to the structures around and supporting the teeth.

periodontitis Inflammation of the area around a tooth.

periosteum The thin fibrous outer layer of a bone.

peristalsis The wave-like squeezing movements of the intestines by which they propel their contents.

peritoneal dialysis A DIALYSIS process for removing poisons or other harmful substances from the patient's blood by circulating fluid through the cavity enclosed by the PERITONEUM.

peritoneum A thin membrane lining the inside of the abdominal cavity and folded closely over the abdominal organs.

peritonitis Inflammation of the PERITONEUM.

peritonsillar abscess The medical term for QUINSY.

pernicious anaemia Anaemia characterized by a fall in the number of red blood cells. The formation of these cells depends on the presence in the diet of an adequate amount of vitamin B_{12} and on its proper absorption by the intestines. In turn the absorption depends on the presence of a substance called the 'intrinsic factor' which is secreted by the lining of the stomach. For unexplained reasons the secretion may stop and once this has happened it never corrects itself. Treatment then consists of injections of vitamin B_{12}, which must be given regularly for life.

pernio The medical term for CHILBLAIN.

Perthes' disease OSTEOCHONDRITIS at the upper end of the FEMUR, which becomes deformed, affecting the movement of the hip joint. It occurs in childhood.

pertussis The medical term for WHOOPING COUGH. (See FEVERS OF CHILDHOOD)

pes cavus A foot with an abnormally high longitudinal arch.

pes planus see **flat foot**

pessary 1 A medication held in a solid but soluble gelatin base, to be inserted into the vagina, usually for the treatment of a local infection. **2** A small structure inserted into the vagina to support the uterus in cases of PROLAPSE.

petechia A small coloured spot on the skin caused by a minute haemorrhage under its surface.

petit mal see **epilepsy**

petrissage In MASSAGE a slight pinching and twisting action with the fingers.

-pexy A suffix meaning 'surgical fixation' or 'anchoring' of part of the body, generally by SUTURE.

pH This symbol, followed by a number, expresses the alkalinity or acidity of a solution. pH7 indicates that it is neutral. Numbers above this are alkaline; those below are acid.

phaeochromocytoma A tumour of the ADRENAL GLANDS associated with sudden attacks of high blood pressure.

phagocytes Cells, such as certain LEUCOCYTES, which are able to surround, absorb and destroy bacteria and cellular debris in the blood.

phalanx Any bone or segment of a toe or finger.

phallus The penis.

phantom limb The awareness of pain or other sensation in the lost part after an amputation as if it were still present.

pharmacology The study of drugs and their effects.

pharmacopoeia An authoritative publication describing drugs and their use.

pharynx The rear wall of the throat, extending from the back of the nose to the LARYNX and the beginning of the OESOPHAGUS.

phenylketonuria A rare inherited disease in which the body cannot breakdown one PROTEIN component found in many foods. The accumulation of this chemical to abnormal levels in the blood interferes with brain development and the child becomes a mental defective.

   The condition can be spotted by routine urine tests and, if the disease is detected, it can be treated by a restricted diet.

phimosis Abnormal tightness of the FORESKIN so that it cannot be retracted back from the GLANS PENIS.

phlebitis Inflammation of a vein.

phlebography ANGIOGRAPHY of a vein.

phlebotomy see **venesection**

phlyctenula A small blister or ulcer on the CORNEA or CONJUNCTIVA.

phobia A neurosis in which the patient has a persistent and irrational fear of some object or situation.

phocomelia A congenital defect of limbs, which fail to develop and may be only rudimentary.

phonocariogram A graphic record of heart sounds.

photophobia Abnormal sensitivity of the eyes to light.

photosensitivity Abnormal sensitivity of the skin to sunlight.

phrenic Relating to the DIAPHRAGM.

phthisis An old term for: **1** Wasting of the body.
2 Tuberculosis.

physiology The study of the functions and chemical
processes in the body.

physiotherapy Treatment using physical methods
including exercise, MASSAGE, electricity, heat and water.

pia mater The innermost of the three MENINGES which
cover the brain and SPINAL CORD.

pica A craving to eat substances which are unsuitable as
food, such as coal or plaster.

pigeon chest A deformity of chest characterized by the
abnormal prominence of the breastbone.

piles see **haemorrhoids**

pilonidal sinus A small abnormal pit in the skin at the base
of the spine containing hairs. It may give trouble by
becoming infected.

pineal gland A small structure within the brain believed to
influence sexual development and to control the
day-and-night biological rhythms.

pink disease A disease in small children, causing redness
and swelling of hands and feet, loss of weight,
PHOTOPHOBIA and sweating. It is considered to have been
due to the presence of mercury (no longer used) in
teething powders.

pinna The outer, visible part of the ear.

pisiform One of the CARPAL bones. (See SKELETON)

pituitary gland

pituitary gland An ENDOCRINE GLAND attached to the base
of the brain and composed of two lobes. Its front lobe
secretes several HORMONES which regulate growth and
bone formation, and affect the ADRENAL GLANDS, the
OVARIES and TESTES, the THYROID GLAND, and milk
production in the breasts. The rear lobe releases two
hormones, one of which regulates the amount of urine
produced by the kidneys, the other playing a part in the
contraction of the UTERUS and of the milk ducts in the
breasts.

pityriasis rosea A generally mild skin rash consisting of
small scattered oval spots and lasting a few weeks.

placebo An inactive preparation prescribed to a patient for
its psychological effect.

placenta The organ which develops within the uterus
during pregnancy to allow nourishment to pass from the
mother's blood to that of the FOETUS; the afterbirth.

placenta praevia A condition in which the placenta lies
lower than usual and is situated near or across the
opening of the uterus. It may cause bleeding before or
during labour and obstruct the delivery of the baby.

plague A severe infection affecting rats and passed to man
by the bites of rat fleas. Epidemics occurred on a massive
scale throughout history, notably in the 14th and 17th
centuries, but attacks are now rare. In the bubonic form
swollen, infected lymph glands (bubos) appear in the
armpits and groins. The pneumonic form can be caught
by one person from another.

plantar Relating to the sole of the foot.

plantar response or **Babinski test** The REFLEX downward bending of the toes when the sole of the foot is stroked hard. The opposite reaction of upward movement indicates some trouble in the nervous system, except in babies when this response is normal.

plaque Any flat area or patch which differs from the surrounding area.

plasma The fluid portion of the blood without the blood cells.

plasmapharesis Removal of blood, separation of its cells and their re-injection into the patient's body in concentrated form in a suitable fluid.

plasmodium A parasite of the type found in MALARIA.

plastic surgery The reconstruction and repair of deformities and the improvement of appearance, including SKIN GRAFTS.

platelets Very small round or oval bodies in the blood which play an essential role in COAGULATION.

–plegia A suffix meaning 'paralysis'.

pleura A double-layered membrane which lies against and covers each lung. (See LUNGS)

pleurisy Inflammation of the PLEURA.

pleurodynia Pain in the muscles between the ribs or pain like that associated with pleurisy. (See also BORNOLM DISEASE)

plumbism Chronic lead poisoning.

Plummer–Vinson's syndrome A condition of anaemia with inflamed tongue and mouth and difficulty in swallowing.

-pnea A suffix meaning 'relating to breathing'.

pneumoconiosis A disease of the lungs which develops from long-continued inhalation of certain particles. Examples are asbestosis, silicosis and byssinosis, from asbestos, silica and cotton dust respectively. Fibrous scar tissue is formed in the lungs and may predispose to chest infections.

pneumo–encephalography ENCEPHALOGRAPHY by means of the injection of air into the ventricles of the brain.

pneumonectomy Surgical removal of a lung.

pneumonia or **pneumonitis** Inflammation of the lungs. (See BRONCHOPNEUMONIA and LOBAR PNEUMONIA)

pneumoperitoneum Air or gas in the cavity bounded by the PERITONEUM.

pneumothorax Air or gas in the space between the layers of the PLEURA, causing pressure on and partial collapse of the lung.

podagra Gout.

poliomyelitis A VIRUS infection which attacks the SPINAL CORD and causes paralysis, especially of the limbs and sometimes of the breathing muscles. (See FEVERS OF CHILDHOOD)

pollex The thumb.

poly– A prefix meaning 'many' or 'much'.

polyarteritis nodosa A COLLAGEN DISEASE of inflammation of small ARTERIES in various parts of the body. The arteries may become blocked and this will affect the function of the organs they serve, for example, the kidneys and lungs, and also the skin.

polyarthritis Inflammation of several joints.

polycystic kidney The formation of several CYSTS in the kidney.

polycythaemia A condition marked by an abnormally high number of ERYTHROCYTES in the blood. It may sometimes develop as a response to sustained breathing difficulties, as in heart or lung diseases, or through living in the rarefied atmosphere of high altitudes. The extra erythrocytes can carry more oxygen to the tissues.

polycythaemia vera A disease characterized by an excessive number of ERYTHROCYTES in the blood, which thicken it, causing difficulties in circulation and the risk of THROMBOSIS.

polydactylism The presence of extra fingers or toes on the hands or feet.

polymyalgia rheumatica A disease associated with pain in and stiffness of the muscles in several parts of the body.

polyp A small growth or projection from a MUCOUS MEMBRANE.

polypharmacy Prescribing or giving many drugs at the same time. The term generally implies excessive medication.

polyposis The formation of many POLYPS.

polyuria The passing of an excessive amount of urine.

pompholyx A rash with small vesicles on the hands or feet causing irritation.

popliteal Relating to the area behind the knee.

porphyria A condition in which porphyrins, a chemical component of HAEMOGLOBIN, are excreted in the urine, colouring it pink or purple or making it darken on exposure to light. It may be CONGENITAL, and is accompanied by PHOTOSENSITIVITY. It may appear in adults as a reaction to sensitivity to some drugs or to an illness and cause abdominal pains, neuritis and mental confusion.

portal hypertension Excessively high pressure in the PORTAL VEIN. It can be caused by abnormalities of the vein or by CIRRHOSIS of the liver.

portal vein The vein which carries blood from the intestines and stomach, and from associated organs like the spleen and pancreas, to the LIVER. In this way digested materials are passed to the liver for processing.

post- A prefix meaning 'after' or 'behind'.

postmaturity The condition of an infant at birth when pregnancy has extended unduly beyond its usual time. Difficulties may arise from the size of the baby at delivery and from the fact that the PLACENTA has not been able to keep pace with the nourishment required by the baby.

post-mortem examination see **autopsy**

postpartum Relating to the period immediately after childbirth.

postpartum haemorrhage Abnormally heavy bleeding from the uterus immediately after delivery.

Pott's fracture Fracture of the lower end of the FIBULA, which may involve DISLOCATION of or damage to the ankle joint.

poultice A hot, thick, medicated dressing applied as a COUNTERIRRITANT.

P.P.H. An abbreviation for POSTPARTUM HAEMORRHAGE.

p.r. An abbreviation for per rectum – diagnostic examination by palpation or inspection of the rectum.

pre- A prefix meaning 'before' and relating to time or the position.

prefrontal leucotomy see **leucotomy**

prematurity The condition of a baby born well before the usual term of pregnancy and therefore not fully developed.

premedication Drugs administered to a patient to prepare him for any special medical process, especially sedation before being taken for an operation.

premenstrual tension Feelings of heaviness and emotional upset experienced by some women in the few days immediately before the onset of their menstrual periods.

premolar teeth see **teeth**

prepatellar bursitis see **housemaid's knee**

prepuce The foreskin of the penis.

presbyacusis Progressive hearing loss in old age.

presbyopia Reduction in the power to focus the eyes fully in old age.

presentation

presentation That part of the baby which will be born first, i.e. the part that passes first into to the birth canal. (See also LIE)

pressure sore An ULCER of the skin caused by sustained pressure. (See also BED SORE)

priapism Persistent erection of the penis.

prickly heat Blockage of the sweat glands with the formation of small skin blisters and a rash.

primary Describes an abnormal condition which subsequently causes another, or secondary, abnormality.

primigravida A woman who is pregnant for the first time.

primipara A woman who has borne one child.

p.r.n. A prescription indication meaning 'as and when required' – the initials of the Latin words 'pro re nata'.

procidentia PROLAPSE of the womb.

proctalgia Pain in the RECTUM.

proctalgia fugax A condition giving sudden, severe cramp-like attacks of PROCTALGIA.

proctitis Inflammation of the RECTUM.

proctology The branch of medicine concerned with diseases of the RECTUM and ANUS.

proctoscope An illuminated SPECULUM for examining the RECTUM.

progeria A rare condition of premature ageing and senility in a child.

progesterone One of the HORMONES secreted by the ovaries and also by the PLACENTA. It plays a part in the control of the menstrual cycle and in safeguarding the normal progress of a pregnancy.

progestogen Any preparation having an effect similar to that of PROGESTERONE.

prognosis Forecast of the likely course and result of a disease.

prolactin A HORMONE formed by the PITUITARY GLAND which stimulates the production of milk.

prolapse The falling or displacement of an organ or structure, for example, a prolapsed INTERVERTEBRAL DISC or a prolapsed UTERUS.

pronation Turning the forearm so that the palm faces backwards or downwards.

prone Lying down face downwards.

prophylaxis The prevention of disease.

proprioceptive Relating to the nerve elements which give information about movement or position of parts of the body.

prostaglandins A group of chemicals present in many parts of the body. Their varied actions include an effect on the contraction of the uterus, roles in pain and inflammation, and the ability to lower the blood pressure.

prostatectomy Surgical removal of all or part of the PROSTATE GLAND.

prostate gland In the male a gland below the bladder and surrounding the first part of the URETHRA. It secretes part of the SEMEN.

prostatitis Inflammation of the PROSTATE GLAND.

prosthesis Any artificial replacement for a part of the body, for example, a glass eye or an artificial leg.

proteins Complex chemical compounds which are essential to all living matter. They are formed by different combinations of less complex chemicals.

proteinuria Abnormal excess of PROTEINS in the urine.

protozoa (singular, *protozoon*) Simple, primitive microscopic forms of life consisting of single-celled ORGANISMS.

proximal Describing a position relatively closer to the centre of the body. (Compare DISTAL)

prurigo A chronic condition of the skin with formation of itching red PAPULES.

pruritus Itching.

pruritus ani Itching, generally with a rash, around the ANUS.

pruritus vulvae Itching, generally with a rash, around the VULVA.

pseudarthrosis The formation of a 'false joint' where the two broken ends of a bone fracture do not unite but heal separately.

pseudocyesis The appearance of symptoms of pregnancy in a woman who is not pregnant.

psittacosis A pneumonia-like disease transmitted by man from birds, especially parrots and budgerigars.

psoriasis A skin disease characterized by the formation of red patches covered with small white or silvery scales.

psychiatry The branch of medicine concerned with mental and emotional disorders.

psychoanalysis A method of treating certain mental illnesses by enabling the patient to discover for himself suppressed and unconscious fears or memories which are causing his present troubles. Their emergence into, and recognition by, his conscious mind may liberate the patient from his illness.

psychoneurosis see **neurosis**

psychopath Someone whose behaviour is antisocial, irresponsible and frequently abnormally aggressive.

psychosis A mental illness of such severity that the patient loses his sense of reality or any INSIGHT into his state, and may develop DELUSIONS or HALLUCINATIONS. (Compare NEUROSIS)

psychosomatic disease A disease with physical features but originating in mental or emotional factors.

psychotherapy Psychological (as opposed to physical) treatment of mental conditions.

ptosis 1 A PROLAPSE. **2** (Of the eyelid) drooping.

ptyalism The excretion of an excessive amount of SALIVA.

puberty The stage in life in which an individual attains sexual maturity.

pubis The bone forming one half of the front of the pelvis. (See SKELETON)

puerperium The period of time immediately following childbirth, variously assessed as between two and four weeks.

pulmonary Relating to the lung.

pulmonary embolism The blocking by an EMBOLUS of one of the major ARTERIES of the lungs. If the artery is relatively small the symptoms include pain, coughing and later bloodstained SPUTUM. When a large artery is involved the condition is serious, with very severe pain, breathlessness and SHOCK.

pulmonary emphysema An unnatural and permanent distension of the ALVEOLI of the lungs. It can follow some chronic infections of the lungs and airways. Damage to the alveoli impairs the efficiency of their function, and the distension reduces the breathing movements of the chest wall; the patient is short of breath.

pulmonectomy Surgical removal of a lung.

pulp The soft tissue inside a tooth, with blood and nerve supply. (See TEETH)

pulse The palpable pressure wave in an artery, caused by the thrust of blood pumped out of the heart at each beat.

pupil The circular opening in the centre of the IRIS, through which the light enters the eye. Normally it contracts in bright light and in the ACCOMMODATION of looking at close objects.

purpura A spontaneous BRUISE formation on the skin due to some abnormality of the blood or its vessels.

purulent Containing pus.

pus A liquid, generally yellow in colour, produced by INFLAMMATION and INFECTION. It contains LEUCOCYTES, living and dead BACTERIA, and remnants of damaged TISSUES.

pustule A small skin blister with pus.

p.v. Abbreviation for 'per vaginam' – gynaecological examination by palpation or inspection of the vagina.

pyaemia A SEPTICAEMIA with pus or infected clots in the blood, generally producing abscesses in different parts of the body.

pyelitis Inflammation of the pelvis of the kidney.

pyelonephritis Inflammation of the pelvis and of the substance of the kidney.

pyloric stenosis A narrowing of the PYLORUS, interfering with the passage of food from the stomach. In some young babies this condition may produce sudden and violent attacks of vomiting.

pylorus The opening at the end of the stomach through which food enters the duodenum. (See DIGESTIVE TRACT)

pyo- A prefix meaning 'pus'.

pyogenic Producing PUS.

pyorrhoea A discharge of pus, especially in relation to infection of the gums.

pyrexia Fever.

pyridoxine Vitamin B_6. (See VITAMINS)

q.d.s. A prescription indication meaning 'four times a day' – the initials of the Latin words 'quater in die sumendus'.

Q

Q-fever An infectious pneumonia-like illness caused by microbes carried by sheep, goats or cattle. It can be transmitted by ticks or through contaminated dust or food.

q.i.d. see **q.d.s.**

q.s. A prescription indication meaning 'a sufficiency, enough of' – the initials of the Latin words 'quantum sufficiat'. The quantity is left to the dispenser's discretion.

quadriplegia Paralysis of all four limbs.

quarantine Isolation of people suspected of having an infectious disease until the time when they can no longer pass it on to others.

quartan Occurring every fourth day.

quickening The first feeling which a pregnant woman has of the movements of the foetus in the womb. This is generally between the 18th and the 22nd week of pregnancy.

quinsy An ABSCESS in the TONSILS and the surrounding tissues.

R **R** A prescription indication to the dispenser: it instructs him to take and prepare the medicaments which follow. It is an abbreviation for the Latin word 'recipe'.

rabies or **hydrophobia** A severe virus disease caught from the bite or lick of infected animals such as dogs, cats, foxes or bats. After an incubation period varying from ten days to many weeks, it attacks the nervous system. Symptoms include paralysis of the breathing muscles and painful constriction of throat muscles on swallowing or drinking: hence the alternative name of hydrophobia –

'fear of water'. The final stages are marked by convulsions and coma. Investigations and treatment should be initiated as soon as possible after any potentially dangerous bite.

rachitis Rickets.

radiation sickness Illness caused by undue exposure to IONIZING RADIATION, such as X-rays, or that resulting from a nuclear explosion or leakage.

radical mastectomy Surgical excision of a breast and of some of the underlying muscles and associated lymph glands in the AXILLA.

radioactive Emitting electromagnetic radiation by spontaneous changes in the atoms of which it is composed.

radiography The taking of radiographs, X-ray pictures, to assist diagnosis.

radioisotopes Radioactive ISOTOPES.

radiology The diagnostic and therapeutic use of radioactive materials, including X-rays.

radiotherapy The treatment of disease by means of radioactive rays, including X-RAYS.

radius A bone in the forearm. (See SKELETON)

rale An abnormal sound heard in the lungs on AUSCULTATION, indicating constriction of or excessive secretions in the air tubes.

ranula A cyst which develops on the underside of the tongue or on the floor of the mouth. It is generally due to the blockage of a duct from a small SALIVARY GLAND.

rat-bite fever Infection from the bite of a rodent. It produces inflammation at the point of the bite, fever and swollen LYMPH GLANDS.

Raynaud's disease A condition in which the arteries at the extremities (fingers, nose, ears, etc.) narrow in spasm and temporarily restrict their blood supply, causing them to become cold and turn white.

R.B.C. An abbreviation for red blood cell (ERYTHROCYTE).

rectocoele Protrusion of part of the RECTUM into the VAGINA.

rectum The final section of the large intestine, leading to the anus. (See DIGESTIVE TRACT)

red blood cell see **erythrocyte**

reducible Describes a HERNIA whose protrusion can be temporarily corrected by manipulation and pressure and without an operation.

reduction Restoration of a dislocated joint, fractured bone or hernia to its correct position by surgery or by manipulation.

referred pain Pain which is felt not at its site of origin but, because of interconnecting nerve paths, at some other point in the body.

reflex An action which takes place automatically without direction from the conscious mind. Examples are the jerking away of the hand after an unexpected pinprick on the finger or the upwards kick of the leg in the doctor's knee jerk test.

Before reaching the brain, at spinal cord level the impulses carrying sensation trigger off the nerve which stimulates the reflex movement. (See also CONDITIONED REFLEX)

regional enteritis, regional ileitis or **Crohn's disease** Inflammation and thickening of the wall of one section of the intestine, often the ileum, with narrowing of the space within. (See DIGESTIVE TRACT)

rehabilitation Restoring a patient to fitness and self-sufficiency after a severe illness or injury. This procedure includes physiotherapy and, if necessary, training for a new and suitable occupation.

Reiter's disease A feverish illness with URETHRITIS, CONJUNCTIVITIS and ARTHRITIS as its main features.

relapse The increase in severity of a disease after an apparent improvement.

relapsing fever An infectious disease transmitted by infected lice or ticks, and characterized by intermittent bouts of fever.

remission Diminution of the severity of a disease.

renal Relating to the kidney.

renal colic Painful COLIC of the URETER due to obstruction by a CALCULUS from the kidney.

renal hypertension High blood pressure associated with disease of the kidneys.

rep. A prescription indication meaning 'repeat'. For example, 'rep. mist.', an abbreviation for the Latin 'repetatur mistura', means 'repeat the mixture'.

repression In psychiatry the rejection from the conscious mind of unpleasant memories and ideas, which may then lie dormant and SUBCONSCIOUS.

reproductive system, female (see opposite)

reproductive system, male (see page 200)

retention of urine Inability to pass urine owing to blockage of the URETHRA. In men this is commonly due to enlargement of the PROSTATE GLAND.

reticulo–endothelial system The name given to the cells scattered about in various tissues of the body, which have the ability to absorb and destroy bacteria and other foreign invaders. They also produce specific ANTIBODIES.

retina The light-sensitive layer at the back of the eye on which the incoming light rays are focused.

retinal detachment Separation of part of the RETINA from its attachment to the inside of the eyeball. This may follow a blow, but sometimes happens spontaneously.

retinitis Inflammation of the retina.

retinoblastoma A tumour of the eye arising from the RETINA.

retinopathy Any disease or disorder of the RETINA.

retroflexion of the uterus The bending back, away from its usual position, of the upper part of the uterus. (Compare RETROVERSION OF THE UTERUS)

retrolental fibroplasia Proliferation of tissue within the EYE behind the lens, causing blindness. It happened to newborn babies who received excessive and prolonged administration of oxygen.

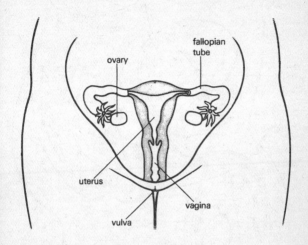

The female internal genital organs. The front of the pelvis has been cut away to show the vagina behind it.

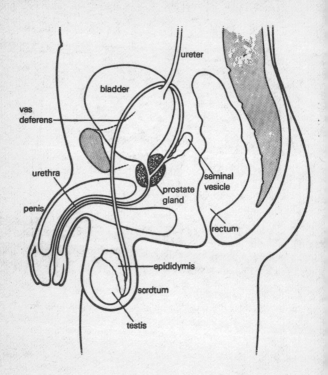

The male genital organs

retroversion of the uterus The sloping back, away from its usual position, of the whole of the uterus. (Compare RETROFLEXION OF THE UTERUS)

Rhesus factor The Rhesus factor (see BLOOD GROUPS) is of importance in the case of a Rhesus positive baby who is born to a Rhesus negative woman. If the woman had in the past received Rhesus positive blood in a transfusion or had in a previous pregnancy carried a Rhesus positive baby then she could have developed in her own blood ANTIBODIES to the Rhesus factor.

In this subsequent pregnancy or labour some of her blood, with these antibodies, may pass into the baby's bloodstream and damage its red blood cells causing ERYTHROBLASTOSIS FOETALIS.

rheumatic fever A disease characterized by fever and by inflammation and swelling arising and subsiding in various large joints and affecting other parts, including the valves of the heart. The joints eventually recover but the heart sometimes remains damaged. The condition appears to be an ALLERGIC reaction to a preceding throat infection caused by STREPTOCOCCI.

rheumatism A term used unspecifically of various kinds of muscle pains and inflammation of the joints.

rheumatoid arthritis A CHRONIC inflammatory disease of the joints, the feet, hands and wrists being particularly affected. In time many cases become less severe but some worsen, causing swelling of the joints with stiffness and deformity. It is considered one of the AUTO-IMMUNE DISEASES.

rhinitis Inflammation of the lining of the nose, for example, as in the common cold.

rhinophyma A form of ROSACEA affecting the nose, which becomes red and swollen.

rhonchus An abnormal harsh noise heard on AUSCULTATION of the chest and caused by partial blockage of the air tubes.

riboflavin Vitamin B_2. (See VITAMINS)

rickets A childhood disease characterized by defective bone formation, showing as a deformity of the ribs and the weight-bearing bones of the legs. It is due to lack of vitamin D resulting from inadequate diet and a deficiency of sunlight (which forms vitamin D in the skin).

rickettsia A genus of small BACTERIA which are transmitted by insects and cause a variety of diseases including TYPHUS.

rigor A sudden attack of violent shivering and a feeling of chill, accompanied by a fast-rising temperature and sweating.

rigor mortis The stiffening and rigidity of the muscles which begin to develop some six hours after death and last about 36 hours.

ringworm see **tinea**

Rinne test A test made with tuning forks to compare the patient's hearing when the fork is held near the ear and when it is held with its handle against the skull by the bone. It compares 'air conduction' and 'bone conduction' of sound and provides information about the condition of different parts of the hearing apparatus of the ear.

ripple bed A bed provided with a mattress divided into sections, each of which is filled with air. An attached pump constantly and gently alters the pressure within the sections. It is used to prevent BED SORES in patients who have to lie still for long periods.

risus sardonicus A tight spasm of muscles of the face producing the impression of grinning.

rodent ulcer A MALIGNANT tumour of the skin, often on the face, in appearance like a raised ulcer. If untreated it may increase in size and cause more damage, but it does not spread to other parts of the body.

Roentgen rays see **X-rays**

Rorschach test A psychological test to assess the patient's personality. He is asked to describe his interpretation of different patterns formed by ink blots.

rosacea A chronic skin disease of the nose and face, with abnormal redness and ACNE.

roseola Any rose-coloured rash.

roseola infantum An acute infection of small children, with fever and enlargement of the lymph glands in the neck. This is followed by the sudden appearance of a rash as the temperature returns to normal.

roundworm A group of PARASITIC worms including HOOKWORM, THREADWORM and the common worm.

-rrage, -rrhoea Suffixes denoting excessive flow of a fluid.

rubella The medical term for GERMAN MEASLES.

rubeola An old name for MEASLES.

Rubin's test A test to show whether both FALLOPIAN TUBES are PATENT, by seeing whether a gas can be passed through them via the uterus.

rupture see **hernia**

S **sacro-iliac joint** The joint between the SACRUM in the centre and the iliac bone at the side of the pelvis. (See SKELETON)

sacrum The central bone at the back of the pelvis and at the base of the backbone. (See SKELETON)

sadism Sexual gratification obtained by inflicting pain or mental suffering on others.

safe period An unreliable calculation of those days in a woman's menstrual cycle when no viable OVUM is present to be fertilized, so that sexual intercourse would not entail the risk of pregnancy.

St Vitus' dance see **Sydenham's chorea**

saliva The fluid secreted into the mouth in order to moisten food and begin the process of digestion.

salivary glands The saliva-secreting glands, located in the cheeks and below the angle of the jaw.

salmonella A group of bacteria which cause diseases like TYPHOID FEVER and PARATYPHOID FEVER and some types of food poisoning.

salpingitis Inflammation of the FALLOPIAN TUBES.

salpingography An X-ray of the FALLOPIAN TUBES, after injecting a CONTRAST MEDIUM, to test whether they are PATENT.

sandfly fever A mild virus infection with influenza-like symptoms, transmitted by the bite of sandflies.

saprophyte Any MICRO-ORGANISM which lives on dead or decaying matter.

sarcoidosis A chronic disease of uncertain origin producing granular points of inflammation in various parts of the body, especially the lungs.

sarcoma A CANCER which arises from CONNECTIVE TISSUE, muscle or bone. (Compare CARCINOMA)

sarcoptes A category of mite, including that found in SCABIES.

satyriasis Excessive sexual desire in a male.

s.c. An abbreviation for SUBCUTANEOUS.

scabies A skin disease with marked itching caused by a mite which burrows under the skin.

scalds BURNS caused by hot fluids or by steam.

scalpel A small surgical knife.

scaphoid 1 One of the small CARPAL bones at the wrist. **2** One of the small TARSAL bones of the foot. (See SKELETON)

scapula The shoulder blade. (See SKELETON)

scarlet fever or **scarlatina** An acute infection caused by a strain of STREPTOCOCCUS, producing a sore throat, fever and a scarlet rash.

Schick test A test to determine a person's IMMUNITY to DIPHTHERIA. A very small dose of diphtheria TOXIN is injected into the skin. The development over the next few days of a certain type of inflammation at the point of the injection indicates absence or insufficiency of diphtheria ANTITOXIN in the body to protect against infection.

schistosomiasis or **bilharziasis** A parasitic tropical disease caused by the larvae of flukes which penetrate the skin of people walking or bathing in contaminated water. The flukes settle mainly in the veins of the bladder and intestines and lay eggs, causing irritation and bleeding in these organs. The eggs pass out with the stools and urine. In areas of low hygiene they may then reach water deposits, where in turn water snails are infested, from which a new set of larvae develop.

schizoid Relating to SCHIZOPHRENIA.

schizophrenia A form of PSYCHOSIS in which the patient becomes inert and withdrawn from emotional personal contact and many forms of reality. He may suffer from DELUSIONS and develop PARANOIA. Some schizophrenics may have bouts of wild excitement.

sciatica Pain along the back of the thigh and extending down the back of the leg. It can have several causes, including those conditions affecting the large sciatic nerve, which lies in that region.

scintigram or **scintiscan** A recording of the presence and distribution of radioactive ISOTOPES introduced into the body for a diagnostic test.

sclera The thick, white outer cover of the eyeball. (See EYE)

sclero– A prefix meaning 'hard'.

scleroderma A COLLAGEN DISEASE producing thickening of the skin and other parts of the body, such as the intestinal tract.

sclerosis Abnormal hardening of a tissue or organ.

scoliosis Curvature of the spine to one side.

scorbutic Relating to SCURVY.

scotoma An area of diminished vision or absence of vision in the visual field of an eye.

screening 1 The routine examination of large numbers of people in order to detect diseases in an early stage.
2 Fluoroscopy.

scrofula An old name for TUBERCULOSIS involving the LYMPH GLANDS of the neck.

scrotum The pouch of skin hanging behind the PENIS which contains the TESTES.

scrub typhus see **tsutsugamushi disease**

scruple An old measure of weight equal to 20 GRAINS or about 1.3 grams.

scurvy An illness caused by deficiency of vitamin C – the absence of fresh fruits and vegetables in the diet. It causes bleeding into the skin, from the gums and (accompanied by pain) under the PERIOSTEUM. (See VITAMINS)

sebaceous cyst A CYST in the skin formed by a blocked and distended SEBACEOUS GLAND filled with sebum.
Sometimes it becomes infected but is generally harmless. If it becomes big and unsightly it can easily be surgically removed.

sebaceous glands The small oil-secreting glands of the skin, each one of which is usually associated with a HAIR FOLLICLE. The oil, or sebum, secreted is a protective lubricant for the skin.

seborrhoea Excessive secretion of sebum from the SEBACEOUS GLANDS.

sebum see **sebaceous glands**

secondaries New MALIGNANT tumours which have developed from the spread of an initial, or primary, tumour.

secondary Describes an abnormal condition which arises as a consequence of another earlier, or primary, condition. (See also AMENORRHOEA)

secretion The production of a substance by a gland or the substance produced.

sedative A drug used for calming or quietening.

sedimentation rate see **erythrocyte sedimentation rate**

semen The fluid ejaculated from the penis by the male.

semicircular canals Three fluid-filled horseshoe-shaped canals within the inner EAR. They are in different planes and register not hearing but position and movement of the head.

semilunar One of the CARPAL bones. (See SKELETON)

semilunar cartilage see **meniscus**

seminal fluid Semen.

seminal vesicle One of two small organs behind the prostate. It secretes fluid which forms the main component of SEMEN. (See REPRODUCTIVE SYSTEM, MALE)

seminoma A MALIGNANT tumour of the TESTIS.

sensory nerve see **nerve**

sepsis The presence in the bloodstream or in the tissues of harmful BACTERIA or their TOXINS.

septicaemia A disease caused by the presence of large numbers of rapidly multiplying bacteria in the bloodstream; blood poisoning.

sequestrum A fragment of dead bone which has become separated from the rest of a diseased bone.

serology The study of SERUM; in particular tests with serum based on the presence of ANTIBODIES.

serum 1 The clear fluid which remains from blood after clotting has taken place. **2** Another name for ANTISERUM.

serum sickness A HYPERSENSITIVITY reaction, with fever, URTICARIA and joint pains, which develops some days after an injection of ANTISERUM.

sesamoid bone A small nodular bone sometimes present within the substance of a TENDON.

sex-linked Relating to a feature inheritable with the sex of the individual. Its GENE is on the X CHROMOSOME.

shaking palsy An old name for PARKINSON'S DISEASE.

shingles An illness caused by the virus of CHICKEN POX. It can arise many years after an attack of chicken pox. The virus, having remained inactive in the body, suddenly causes inflammation of a NERVE, accompanied by pain. This is followed a few days later by skin blisters along the area served by the nerve. In some cases the pain may persist long after the illness has subsided.

shock In medical terminology a dangerous failing of the heart and circulation which can follow heavy bleeding, extensive injury, bruises, burns, severe fractures, rapid fluid loss as caused by severe sweating or diarrhoea, some BACTERIAL blood infections, heart attacks and PULMONARY EMBOLISM.

shock therapy In psychiatry the treatment of certain conditions by causing convulsions or inducing a coma in the patient by means of drugs or electricity.

short sightedness Difficulty in focusing on objects at a distance, although perception of objects close at hand may be good.

shunt A passage between two channels of fluid, for example blood vessels. In some cases of congenital HYDROCEPHALUS an artificial shunt is surgically created to drain the excess CEREBROSPINAL FLUID through a plastic tube into the cavity of the PERITONEUM.

sialitis Inflammation of a SALIVARY gland.

sibling One of two or more children having the same parent.

sickle cell anaemia Anaemia from an inherited abnormality of HAEMOGLOBIN causing deformed and fragile ERYTHROCYTES. In severe cases it can produce bleeding, with pain in the joints, abdomen and other parts of the body.

side effect An unwanted effect of a drug in addition to its desired therapeutic effect.

siderosis 1 Deposits of iron in the tissues. **2** A lung disease caused by inhaling dust or vapours containing iron.

sigmoid colon The final part of the large intestine, before the RECTUM. (See DIGESTIVE TRACT)

sigmoidoscope A tubular instrument with a light which is passed through the ANUS and RECTUM to inspect the SIGMOID COLON.

signs What the doctor finds as abnormalities when he examines the patient. (See DIAGNOSIS)

silicosis PNEUMOCONIOSIS caused by inhalation of silica dust.

sinister On the left-hand side.

sino-atrial node Another term for SINO-AURICULAR NODE.

sino-auricular node A nerve centre in the wall of the right AURICLE of the heart, which sends out rhythmic impulses initiating and coordinating the beat of the VENTRICLES.

sinus 1 A cavity in the body, in particular the nasal sinuses within the skull bones around the nose, containing air and opening into the nose. **2** An abnormal passage from an infected part, leading to the surface and allowing pus to escape through it.

sinusitis Inflammation of the lining of the sinuses of the nose.

situs inversus A congenital condition in which the organs of the body are transposed, as if in a mirror image. Thus, the spleen is on the right and the liver on the left of the abdomen. In itself it has no detrimental effect on health.

sinus node Another term for SINO-AURICULAR NODE.

sinus rhythm The normal heart beat rhythm, controlled by the SINO-AURICULAR NODE. (See HEART)

skeleton (see pages 212–214)

skin graft The transplanting of a piece of skin from one part of a patient's body to cover a defect in another part.

s.l.e. An abbreviation for systemic LUPUS ERYTHEMATOSUS.

skeleton

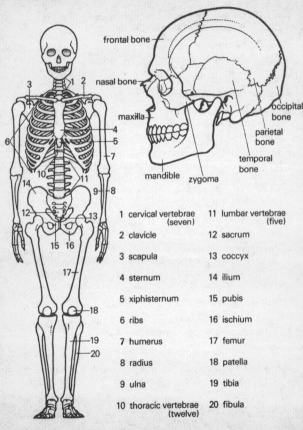

frontal bone

nasal bone

maxilla

mandible   zygoma

occipital bone

parietal bone

temporal bone

1 cervical vertebrae (seven)	11 lumbar vertebrae (five)
2 clavicle	12 sacrum
3 scapula	13 coccyx
4 sternum	14 ilium
5 xiphisternum	15 pubis
6 ribs	16 ischium
7 humerus	17 femur
8 radius	18 patella
9 ulna	19 tibia
10 thoracic vertebrae (twelve)	20 fibula

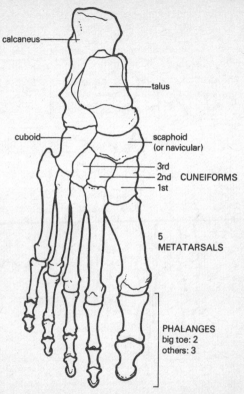

calcaneus

talus

cuboid

scaphoid
(or navicular)

3rd
2nd CUNEIFORMS
1st

5
METATARSALS

PHALANGES
big toe: 2
others: 3

The bones of the right foot seen from above.

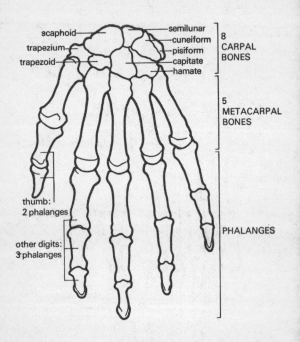

The bones of the left hand seen from above.

sleeping sickness An African form of TRYPANOSOMIASIS, transmitted by the bite of the tsetse fly. It may cause severe inflammation of the brain and spinal cord, with great apathy and drowsiness in the patient or, in some cases, agitation.

sleepy sickness see **encephalitis lethargica**

slipped disc see **intervertebral disc**

slough Dead tissue which becomes separate from the healthy tissue around it.

smallpox An acute and highly CONTAGIOUS virus infection. It begins with fever, severe aching, headaches and vomiting. A rash of pink spots follows, which is more profuse on the face and limbs than on the trunk. The spots become PUSTULES and after healing may leave deep scars (pockmarks).

smear A small quantity of material prepared for microscopic examination by being spread thinly on a glass microscope slide.

smegma A thick secretion which forms under the FORESKIN.

soft sore see **chancroid**

solar plexus A network of nerves behind the stomach. Its branches reach various abdominal organs including the stomach and intestines.

somatic Relating to the body, as opposed to the mind.

somnambulism Sleepwalking.

soporific A drug which induces sleep.

s.o.s. A prescription indication meaning 'if necessary' – the initials of the Latin words 'si opus sit'. This usually implies that the drug is to be administered only once.

souffle A soft blowing sound sometimes heard on AUSCULTATION of the heart.

spastic 1 Characterized by spasms or tightness of muscle, generally caused by abnormality in the nervous control of the muscle. **2** See CEREBRAL PALSY.

spatula A small, flat, blunt tool used for mixing substances or for depressing the tongue when examining the throat.

speculum An instrument inserted into a body orifice or cavity which distends it and allows it to be inspected.

speech therapy Treatment designed to overcome difficulties in speech and communication. These include such defects as stammering and loss of power of speaking, reading or writing after brain damage or as a result of congenital conditions.

spermatic cord A cord-like structure suspending the TESTIS within the SCROTUM, and holding the duct of the TESTIS, blood and lymph vessels, and muscle fibres.

spermatozoa (singular, *spermatozoon*) The male reproductive cells.

sphenoid bone One of two bones of the skull forming part of the eye socket. (See SKELETON)

sphincter A muscular ring which closes a natural passage, for example, at the ANUS.

sphygmomanometer An instrument for measuring blood pressure.

spica A bandage applied so that its successive turns cross each other; a figure-of-eight bandage.

spina bifida A congenital defect in the vertebral column. In one or more VERTEBRAE the bony area behind and enclosing the SPINAL CORD fails to form completely. The cord and its membranes may bulge into the gap.

spinal canal The hollow formed by the VERTEBRAE through which the SPINAL CORD runs.

spinal cord The column of nerve tissue which extends from the base of the brain down the central cavity of the backbone or VERTEBRAL COLUMN.

spine The VERTEBRAL COLUMN.

spirochaetes Spiral-shaped bacteria. Many forms are harmless but others can cause such different conditions as VINCENT'S ANGINA, WEIL'S DISEASE and SYPHILIS.

spleen An organ on the left side of the upper part of the abdomen. Part of the RETICULO-ENDOTHELIAL SYSTEM, it plays a role in developing IMMUNITIES, and in the formation of blood and the breakdown of old blood cells.

splenectomy Surgical removal of the SPLEEN.

splenic anaemia or **Banti's disease** A condition in which there is enlargement of the SPLEEN, ANAEMIA, CIRRHOSIS of the liver and obstruction of the PORTAL VEIN.

splen(o)- A prefix meaning 'relating to the spleen.'

splenomegaly Abnormal enlargement of the SPLEEN.

spondylitis Inflammation of the vertebrae (see VERTEBRAL COLUMN). Ankylosing spondylitis is a form which generally affects young males and gradually causes stiffness of the spine.

spondylosis OSTEOARTHRITIS of the VERTEBRAE.

spore 1 The seed of a fungus. **2** In some bacteria, such as those of tetanus or anthrax, a variation of their usual form which enables them to survive adverse conditions and remain alive until the circumstances (temperature or moisture) become favourable for a return to their ordinary active form.

spotted fever 1 MENINGOCOCCAL MENINGITIS. **2** A term used to cover various infections caused by RICKETTSIA.

sprain Damage to a joint caused by a twist or wrench, with some tearing of the ligaments. (Compare STRAIN)

sprue A disease with diarrhoea, anaemia and weight loss caused by a deficiency in absorption of vitamins and fats by the intestinal tract. 'Tropical sprue' is found in Asia and America. 'Non-tropical sprue' is similar to the coeliac disease of children.

sputum Matter coughed up from the lungs and airways; phlegm. This generally means particles of MUCUS discharge, with some pus, the result of inflammation.

squint Failure of the eyes to point in the same direction, caused by a defect in one or more muscles which move the eyeballs.

stapedectomy The surgical removal of the STAPES and the attachment of an artificial replacement as treatment for OTOSCLEROSIS.

stapes One of the three small bones which transmit soundwaves within the EAR.

staphylococcus A coccus form of BACTERIA, whose minute spherical bodies group to form clusters.

stasis A reduction or cessation in the flow of a body fluid, as, for example, blood.

stat. A prescription indication meaning 'immediately'; the drug to be administered at once. It is an abbreviation for the Latin word 'statim'.

status asthmaticus An attack of ASTHMA which persists an abnormally long time.

status epilepticus An abnormally prolonged attack, or a succession of attacks, of EPILEPSY.

steatorrhoea The passing of excessive fat in the faeces.

Stein-Leventhal syndrome A condition in women of reduced or absent periods, enlarged OVARIES and failure of OVULATION. Obesity and HIRSUTISM are sometimes features.

stenosis Narrowing of a body passage or opening.

stereognosis The ability to assess by touch the shape and nature of objects.

sterile 1 Unable to produce offspring. 2 Free from living micro-organisms.

sternum The breastbone. (See SKELETON)

steroids A large group of chemical compounds including vitamin D, bile acids and many hormones. The term is often used to mean CORTICOSTEROIDS.

stethoscope A doctor's instrument used for AUSCULTATION.

Stevens-Johnson's syndrome An illness of severe ERYTHEMA MULTIFORME, with fever and inflammation of the eye, mouth and genital areas.

stigma (plural, *stigmata*) Any physical or mental abnormality characteristic of a disease and therefore helpful as pointer to diagnosis.

Still's disease A form of RHEUMATOID ARTHRITIS in children. It is generally characterized by severe symptoms but clears up fully.

Stokes–Adams attack Sudden unconsciousness, with loss of pulse beat, occurring in someone with a HEART BLOCK.

stoma An opening into a cavity or area, for example, a deliberate opening made surgically and maintained to drain fluid away from a part of the body.

stomach The enlarged part of the DIGESTIVE TRACT between the end of the OESOPHAGUS and the beginning of the DUODENUM. It secretes hydrochloric acid and PEPSIN and also the 'intrinsic factor'. (See PERNICIOUS ANAEMIA)

stomat- A prefix meaning 'relating to the mouth'.

stomatitis Inflammation of the inside of the mouth.

stools The FAECES discharged from the bowels.

strabismus A squint.

strain Overstretching of and damage to a muscle. (Compare SPRAIN)

strangulated Describes a part of the body caught tightly in an opening in such a way as to interfere with its blood supply, for example, a strangulated hernia. The protruding part is tightly squeezed by the edges of the opening from which it emerges.

strangury The passing of urine slowly with pain and difficulty.

streptococcus A coccus form of BACTERIA, whose minute spherical bodies group to form chain patterns.

stria (plural, *striae*) A scar-like pale streak which appears in skin which has become stretched, as in developing obesity.

striae gravidarum The STRIAE or 'stretch marks' which appear on the mother's abdomen or breasts during pregnancy.

stricture An abnormal narrowing of a tubular passage, for example, stricture of the URETHRA by scarring after inflammation.

stridor A hard, high-pitched BREATH SOUND heard on AUSCULTATION of the chest and made by the passage of air past an obstruction.

stroke A sudden disturbance of some brain function due to rupture or blocking of one of the brain's blood vessels. The nature and degree of the disturbance depend on the area of the brain involved. Paralysis or loss of feeling in some part of the body, difficulty in speaking, swallowing or remembering are possible effects.

stroma The tissues forming the supporting and less specialized parts of an organ. (Compare PARENCHYMA)

strongyloides A parasitic worm which can infest the intestines, causing diarrhoea and ulceration of the bowels.

struma An old name for GOITRE.

stump The end of a limb after amputation.

stupor Partial unconsciousness.

stye Infection and abscess formation in a SEBACEOUS GLAND of an eyelid.

sub- A prefix meaning 'beneath' or 'under'.

subacute Describes an illness halfway between CHRONIC and ACUTE.

subacute bacterial endocarditis A bacterial infection attacking the heart valves which have previously been damaged, either because of CONGENITAL factors or as a result of RHEUMATIC FEVER.

subarachnoid haemorrhage Bleeding into the subarachnoid space of the brain. (See MENINGES)

subclavian Relating to the region beneath the CLAVICLE.

subconscious Mental activity which takes place below the level of conscious awareness.

subcostal Relating to the region below the ribs.

subcutaneous Under the skin – usually with reference to injections.

subjective Describes what is perceived or experienced personally by the individual concerned but not by others.

sublimation The unconscious substitution of an acceptable action for an emotional reaction which would be socially unacceptable. This may, for example, take the form of channelling activities into sport to overcome a feeling of violence resulting from frustration in some other part of one's life.

subliminal Describes an event, as a sight or sound, which is of insufficient strength to be consciously appreciated by the senses.

subluxation An incomplete DISLOCATION. The bones concerned have been displaced in the joint, but not fully separated.

submental Below the chin.

submucosa The tissue under a MUCOUS MEMBRANE.

subphrenic Beneath the DIAPHRAGM.

subtotal gastrectomy Surgical removal of part of the stomach.

subungual Beneath a nail.

succussion The splashing sound heard from a cavity containing both air and fluid when the body is shaken.

sudor Sweat.

sulcus A groove or furrow.

superego In psychology that part of the personality which governs the conscience, is concerned with ethics and moral standards, and counterbalances the ID. (See also EGO)

superinfection A new infection which complicates the course of treatment of a primary infection by introducing BACTERIA resistant to that treatment.

supernumary In excess of the normal number, for example, a sixth finger on a hand.

supination Turning the forearm so that the palm faces forwards or upwards.

supine Lying on the back.

suppository A medicated semi-solid preparation to be inserted into the RECTUM.

suppurating Forming or discharging PUS.

supra- A prefix meaning 'over' or 'above'.

suprarenal glands see **adrenal glands**

sural Relating to the calf of the leg.

surgical emphysema Abnormal presence of air in an organ or under the skin. It can follow injury or (rarely) surgical operations.

suture A stitch used in surgery.

sycosis barbae An infection of the HAIR FOLLICLES in the region of the beard; barber's rash.

Sydenham's chorea or **St Vitus' dance** Found in children, this is a temporary condition associated with RHEUMATIC FEVER, producing uncontrolled muscle spasms, and causing grimacing and writhing or jerky movements of the limbs. It is unrelated to HUNTINGDON'S CHOREA. (See also CHOREA)

symbiosis A situation in which two organisms live together in some biological association, for example, as PARASITES or COMMENSALS.

sympathectomy A surgical operation to cut out part of the SYMPATHETIC NERVOUS SYSTEM of nerves in order to reduce, for example, an abnormal spasm of blood vessels.

sympathetic nervous system see **autonomic nervous system**

symptoms What the patient himself feels and notices about his illness. (See DIAGNOSIS)

syncope A fainting.

syndactyly The fusion of two adjacent toes or fingers.

syndrome A group of SIGNS and SYMPTOMS which together form the features of a particular disease.

synovectomy Excision of the SYNOVIAL MEMBRANE.

synovial fluid The fluid which is held within the SYNOVIAL MEMBRANE. It acts as a lubricant in movements of a joint.

synovial membrane The smooth inner lining of a JOINT.

syphilis A VENEREAL DISEASE caused by infection with the bacteria treponema pallidum. The first feature or primary stage, the CHANCRE, appears usually about three weeks after infection, although this is very variable. When the chancre has healed, if the disease remains untreated the secondary stage develops about six weeks later, resulting from the spread of bacteria through the blood to all parts of the body. Rashes, sores and lymph gland swellings may be features. The tertiary stage of an untreated case may appear only many years later, following damage by bacteria to various organs such as the spinal cord (see TABES DORSALIS), the heart, eyes and brain.

syringomyelia An illness in which small fluid-filled cavities develop in the SPINAL CORD. They interfere with the adjacent nerve fibres and cause the patient to lose the sensation of touch and temperature in different parts of his body. In later stages the functions of other nerves may be lost.

systemic Relating to the body as a whole. A drug taken systemically, by mouth or by injection, is distributed throughout the body. (Compare TOPICAL)

systole The phase in each heart beat when the VENTRICLES are contracting and pumping out blood. (Compare DIASTOLE and see also BLOOD PRESSURE)

systolic Relating to the SYSTOLE.

T   **tabes dorsalis** A form of ATAXIA, slowly progressive and a late manifestation (after an interval of 10–20 years) of untreated or inadequately treated SYPHILIS. Damage to nerve fibres in the SPINAL CORD leads to sharp attacks of pain, loss of sense of touch in the legs, loss of balance, difficulty in walking, loss of bladder control and sometimes defects of vision.

tachy- A prefix meaning 'rapid'.

tachycardia A fast pulse rate.

tachypnoea Abnormally fast breathing.

tactile Relating to the sense of touch.

taenia The medical name for some forms of TAPEWORM.

talipes see **club foot**

talus The bone at the ankle joint. (See SKELETON)

tamponade Abnormal compression of part of the body. 'Cardiac tamponade' is compression of the heart caused by the presence of blood within the layers of the PERICARDIUM.

tap A surgical manoeuvre to drain fluid or take a sample of fluid from within some part of the body.

tapeworms Worms with many segments forming a long ribbon shape. They can be caught by eating undercooked beef, pork or fish contaminated with the cystic form of the parasite. The mature worms hang on to the inner surface of the intestines and there can grow to a length of several yards. (See also CYSTICERCUS)

tapotement In MASSAGE a tapping action.

tarsal Relating to the bones of the foot at the ankle.

tarsus 1 The ankle **2** The CARTILAGE plate forming the inner support of an eyelid.

tartar A hard mineral deposit which forms on teeth.

Tay-Sach's disease A form of AMAUROTIC FAMILIAL IDIOCY in infants.

t.d.s. A prescription indication meaning 'three times a day' – the initials of the Latin words 'ter in die sumendus'.

teeth (see pages 228–229)

telangiectasis Small dark red spots on the skin formed by the dilation of blood vessels in the area.

temperature A measure of the degree of heat of a body. The normal temperature range of a healthy person is between 36° and 37°C (97° and 99°F).

temperomandibular joint The joint between the lower jawbone and the side of the skull, just in front of the ear.

temporal Relating to the temple.

temporal arteritis A condition marked by inflammation of the arteries of the temple and the scalp, often associated with pain, headaches and fever. The cause is not fully known.

temporal bone One of two bones, each forming part of the side of the skull in the region of the ear. (See SKELETON)

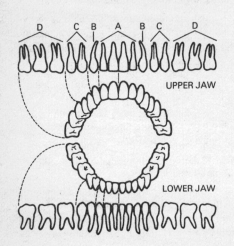

UPPER JAW

LOWER JAW

A: incisors (8)

B: canines (4)

C: premolars (8)

D: molars (12)

Milk teeth begin to erupt about the sixth month and are completely erupted at the end of the second year. There are ten in each jaw, i.e. five teeth in each half-jaw: two incisors, a canine and two molars. They are shed as the permanent teeth erupt. There are 32 permanent teeth altogether, divided equally between the two jaws.

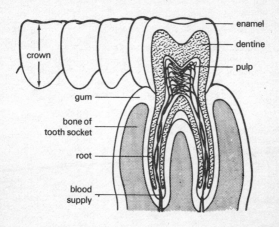

The structure of the teeth

tenderness Pain felt on touch or pressure.

tendinitis Inflammation of a TENDON.

tendon The firm non-elastic band which leads from the end of a muscle to be attached to the bone on which the muscle acts.

tenesmus Painful straining when defecating or urinating.

tennis elbow Tenderness on the outer side of the elbow joint, with pain radiating down the forearm and made worse by gripping and pulling with the hand. It is due to strain on the TENDONS of some forearm muscles after they have been subjected to much action.

teno– A prefix meaning 'relating to a TENDON'.

tenoplasty Repair of a TENDON by PLASTIC SURGERY.

tenosynovitis Inflammation of a TENDON and of the sheath around it. It commonly occurs near the wrist.

tenotomy The surgical cutting of a TENDON.

teratogen Any substance which can cause defects in a developing embryo.

teratoma 1 A tumour containing various elements of foetal tissues. **2** An extremely deformed FOETUS.

terminal Relating to the final period of a fatal disease.

tertian Occurring every third day.

testicles see **testis**

testis (plural, *testes*) One of the two male sex glands lying in the SCROTUM. It produces SPERMATOZOA, the male reproductive cells, and also the HORMONE TESTOSTERONE.

testosterone The HORMONE produced by the TESTES and responsible for the sexual characteristics of the male body.

tetanus Infection from a BACILLUS present in soil, in street dust and in the intestines of animals. In the form of SPORES the bacillus can survive for many years and become active when transmitted to an environment with suitable ANAEROBIC conditions, such as a deep cut or wound. Its TOXIN affects nerves and the spinal cord causing at first muscle stiffness. The early symptom of difficulty in opening the jaw is responsible for the popular name lockjaw. Eventually it produces severe spasms, with convulsions, difficult breathing and even violent rearward arching of the back. Protection by IMMUNIZATION is essential, especially for those active in agriculture and in gardening.

tetany A condition in which muscles are over-excitable, producing cramp, CARPO-PEDAL SPASM or twitching of the face muscles. It has various causes including an abnormally low amount of calcium salts in the blood.

tetralogy of Fallot see **Fallot's tetralogy**

thalamus Part of the brain acting as a relay centre for the nerves from the spine to the CEREBRAL CORTEX.

thalassaemia A HEREDITARY form of anaemia with imperfect HAEMOGLOBIN and thin, fragile ERYTHROCYTES. It occurs mainly in inhabitants of Mediterranean regions.

thenar Relating to the thickened area of the palm at the base of the thumb.

therapy Treatment.

thermo- A prefix meaning 'heat'.

thermography A method of recording pictorially variations in the heat given off by different areas of the body surface. As these depend largely on the circulation of blood in individual underlying parts a departure from the normal can help diagnose various abnormalities, such as tumours.

thermolabile Easily altered by heat.

thiamine Vitamin B_1. (See VITAMINS)

thoracic Relating to the chest.

thoracocentesis PARACENTESIS through the chest wall.

thoracoplasty A surgical operation which removes several ribs to allow the chest wall and the underlying lung to collapse. This was used in the past to allow a lung abscess or cavity to heal.

thoracotomy A surgical operation which involves the opening of the chest wall.

thorax The chest and its contents.

threadworm A small parasitic worm, found in the intestinal tract, particularly the RECTUM.

thrombo- A prefix meaning 'clot'.

thrombo-angiitis obliterans see **Buerger's disease**

thrombocyte Another name for a PLATELET.

thrombocytopenia An abnormally low number of PLATELETS in the blood.

thrombophlebitis Inflammation of a vein, with the formation of a THROMBUS.

thrombosis The formation of a THROMBUS in a blood vessel.

thrombus A blood clot which forms on the inside of a blood vessel or of the heart.

thrush A MONILIA infection in the mouth, producing white patches inside the mouth.

thymus gland A gland-like organ behind the upper part of the breastbone. It produces LYMPHOCYTES and is believed to play an important part in the development of the body's IMMUNITY and AUTO–IMMUNE processes. After childhood it becomes considerably reduced in size.

thyroglossal cyst A CYST in the mid-line of the neck, derived from the persistence of a structure which normally disappears during the development of the FOETUS.

thyroidectomy Surgical removal of all or part of the THYROID GLAND.

thyroid gland An ENDOCRINE GLAND at the base of the neck. It secretes HORMONES necessary for growth and development of the body, and for controlling METABOLISM and also the level of calcium in the blood to ensure the proper development of bones.

thyroiditis Inflammation of the THYROID GLAND.

thyrotoxicosis or **Basedow's disease** A disease due to overactivity of the THYROID GLAND. It produces a goitre, accelerated METABOLISM in the body, loss of weight, fast heart action, mental irritability and sometimes EXOPHTHALMOS.

thyroxine A HORMONE secreted by the THYROID GLAND.

tibia One of the bones in the lower leg. (See SKELETON)

tic A habitual twitch or spasm, sometimes of psychological origin

tic douloureux see **trigeminal neuralgia**

tick A small blood-sucking animal, related to the spider and capable of transmitting various diseases including those caused by RICKETTSIA.

t.i.d. see **t.d.s.**

tinea The name given to several skin diseases caused by fungal infection; ringworm.

tinnitus A sensation of sounds in one or both ears, unrelated to outside noises. Varying from ringing and hissing to roaring, it can have the simplest cause like wax in the ear canal or more serious ones like disturbances of the auditory nerve. Large doses of some drugs, such as aspirin, can cause tinnitus.

tissue Any living matter of one special type designed for a particular function and formed of cells of similar structures, such as fatty tissue, liver tissue or CONNECTIVE TISSUE.

tocopherol Vitamin E. (See VITAMINS)

toilet The cleaning and dressing of a wound.

tomography RADIOGRAPHY of a selected plane in a specific part of the body.

-tomy A suffix meaning 'surgical incision' or 'cutting'.

tongue–tie Restricted movement of the tongue due to abnormal shortness of the membrane which links its lower surface to the floor of the mouth.

tonometry A measure of tension or pressure, for example, that within the eyeball.

tonsil A collection of lymphatic tissue on either side at the back of the throat.

tonsillectomy Surgical removal of the tonsils.

tonsillitis Inflammation of the tonsils.

tooth see **teeth**

tophus A chalky deposit in the skin or elsewhere forming a small lump. It is found with GOUT.

topical Relating to one particular area of the body. A drug is administered topically for its local action, for example, an ointment on a rash or drops in the eye.

torticollis Twisting of the neck caused by contraction of its muscles; wryneck.

tourniquet A band wrapped tightly round a limb to reduce or arrest the blood supply beyond it and to control bleeding. Carefully applied, it is employed in some surgical operations but it should not be used in first aid.

toxaemia Any condition due to the presence of TOXINS in the blood.

toxaemia of pregnancy A condition of pregnancy in which the patient develops ALBUMINURIA, raised BLOOD PRESSURE and retention of water in the body, with OEDEMA of hands and ankles.

toxic goitre see **thyrotoxicosis**

toxin A poisonous substance produced by BACTERIA.

toxo- A prefix meaning 'poison'.

toxoid A TOXIN which has been chemically treated to remove its power to harm, while preserving its ability, if injected, to create IMMUNITY.

toxoplasmosis A disease due to a PROTOZOON PARASITE, toxoplasma, found in many animals including pets. Generally it causes little trouble, but can produce rashes and enlargement of the LYMPH GLANDS. However, if a pregnant woman is infected it can be passed to the foetus with serious results.

trachea A straight tube leading towards the LUNGS from the LARYNX; the windpipe. It divides into a right and left BRONCHUS for the corresponding lungs.

tracheitis Inflammation of the TRACHEA.

tracheo(s)tomy Surgical incision into the TRACHEA to create an opening. It may be carried out as a matter of urgency to relieve obstruction in the airway above it.

trachoma Serious chronic CONJUNCTIVITIS which may lead to blindness as a result of scarring and PANNUS.

traction Pulling or drawing. This can be used to correct deformities caused by dislocations or fractures.

tranquillizer A drug given to calm emotions or to reduce anxiety.

trans- A prefix meaning 'through' or 'across'.

transection The surgical action of cutting across part of the body.

transexual A person who wishes to become a member of the opposite sex.

transference The projection by a patient during PSYCHOANALYSIS of feelings associated with some other authoritative person on to the analyst. The patient then assesses the analyst according to these feelings.

transfusion The transfer of blood from a healthy person into the circulation of a patient.

transillumination The examination and assessment of the condition of an organ by passing a strong light through it.

transplantation The grafting into the body of a TISSUE or ORGAN from another part of the body or from another person's body.

transvestite Someone who obtains sexual pleasure from dressing in the clothing of the opposite sex.

trapezium One of the CARPAL bones. (See SKELETON)

trauma 1 A wound. **2** A severe emotional disturbance.

trematode A parasitic worm; a fluke.

tremor A shaking or trembling of a part of the body.

trephine A surgical instrument used for making a hole in the skull.

trichiasis A condition in which the eyelashes grow inwards towards the eyeball.

trichiniasis or **trichinosis** An illness caused by a parasitic worm and caught by eating undercooked, diseased pork. The larvae may settle in the muscles and produce muscular pains.

tricho-

tricho- A prefix meaning 'hair'.

trichobezoar BEZOAR composed of hair.

trichomonas vaginalis A small PROTOZOON which can infect the VAGINA, causing an irritant discharge.

trichophyton A fungus which tends to attack the hair and nails.

trigeminal nerve The fifth CRANIAL NERVE, it carries sensation to the forehead, face and chin.

trigeminal neuralgia NEURALGIA which affects the TRIGEMINAL NERVE, causing sudden, sharp and severe pains on one side of the face. Sometimes they are triggered off by a quite light touch.

trigger finger A condition characterized by difficulty, and sometimes pain, in straightening a bent finger. Its apparent locking in position can be overcome by effort with a 'snap'. It is due to thickening of a tendon and its sheath.

triquetrum One of the CARPAL bones. (See SKELETON)

trismus Spasm of the jaw muscles, with difficulty in opening the mouth.

trocar and cannula A double instrument used for piercing a hollow organ and draining fluid from it. A sharpened rod (trocar) fits into a tube (cannula) and is withdrawn from it after the organ has been pierced. The cannula remains to allow the fluid to escape.

trochanter The greater and lesser trochanters are bony knobs at the upper end of the femur.

trochlear nerve The fourth CRANIAL NERVE, it supplies the muscles which control the movements of the eyeball.

trophic Relating to nourishment.

tropical sore see **Leishmaniasis**

truss A device worn externally to correct the bulging of a HERNIA and to keep it in place.

trypanosome A PROTOZOAN PARASITE which, in different forms, causes illnesses like SLEEPING SICKNESS in Africa and CHAGAS' DISEASE in South America.

trypanosomiasis Infection by TRYPANOSOMES.

tsutsugamushi disease A form of TYPHUS transmitted by mites and found in Asia and the Pacific area.

tubal pregnancy An ECTOPIC PREGNANCY in the FALLOPIAN TUBE.

tubercle see **tuberculosis**

tuberculin A PROTEIN derived from the bacilli of TUBERCULOSIS but not causing disease.
Sensitivity to it from past or present infection is the basis of the MANTOUX TEST.

tuberculin test A test showing previous or present infection from tuberculosis according to the reaction of the skin at the spot where a small amount of TUBERCULIN is injected into it.

tuberculosis Infection with the tubercle BACILLUS, of which there are two main sorts affecting man. The bovine (cattle) strain is generally transmitted through milk from infected cows. The human strain is usually caught by breathing in invisible droplets of moisture coughed or sneezed out by an infected person.

The tubercle is a resultant small area of inflammation and tissue destruction, forming a mass of 'caseation' or thick pus. This may remain as an infective process which makes a cavity in the tissues. Or it may heal by becoming encased in thick fibrous tissue which hardens by calcification, i.e. deposits of calcium.

'Primary tuberculosis' is infection in someone affected by the bacillus for the first time. Frequently this heals, but the individual has developed sensitivity to the bacillus. 'Post-primary' tuberculosis is a re-activation of the original infection or a re-infection. Primary tuberculosis is very commonly developed early in life in a mild undiagnosed form, which heals without trouble.

tuberous sclerosis A rare congenital condition characterized by firm nodules in the brain and often associated with mental defects, epilepsy, skin lesions and lack of muscle power.

tularaemia An infectious disease affecting wild rodents, such as rabbits, hares and squirrels, but transmissible to men who handle these animals. The illness begins with an ulcer of the skin, followed by fever and pains in the body, and is also characterized by enlarged LYMPH GLANDS.

tumour A swelling, in particular a neoplasm, that is, a growth of cells of one TISSUE forming a mass which has no purpose in the body. A benign tumour does not disseminate and is harmless except that it may cause trouble through pressure and obstruction. A malignant tumour may harm by dissemination in the body or by invasion of other tissues.

tympanic membrane The eardrum.

tympanites see **meterorism**

tympanitis Inflammation of the eardrum.

typhoid fever A bacterial infection of the intestines caused by contaminated food or water. The bacteria are found in the FAECES and sometimes the urine of man. Poor sanitation and the action of flies spread the disease.

The illness is severe with diarrhoea, occasionally constipation, and bloodstained faeces. Sometimes loss of blood is heavy. Recovered patients may become CARRIERS.

typhus A group of related infectious diseases transmitted by lice, tics, fleas and mites. They cause fever with severe prostration, aching in the limbs and the back, rashes and often a form of pneumonia.

ulcer A breach or defect of the skin or MEMBRANE producing an open sore and exposing the tissues beneath.

U

ulcerative colitis ULCERATION and INFLAMMATION of the COLON. A CHRONIC and severe disease, with diarrhoea and the passage of blood and MUCUS. It may be one of the AUTO-IMMUNE DISEASES.

ulna One of the bones of the forearm. (See SKELETON)

ultra– A prefix meaning 'beyond'.

ultrasound Very high pitched sound waves, beyond the range of the human ear. They are used in PHYSIOTHERAPY for the deep warmth produced by their vibrations and are also used in ECHOGRAPHY.

ultraviolet rays Invisible radiation beyond the violet end of the spectrum. It is used for treating certain skin diseases.

umbilical cord The cord containing blood vessels connecting the FOETUS with the PLACENTA and through which it receives nourishment.

umbilical hernia HERNIA at or to the side of the navel.

umbilicus The depression in the centre of the abdomen at the site where the UMBILICAL CORD is attached to the foetus; the navel.

undescended testis A TESTIS which has remained in a foetal situation within the abdomen or at groin level and has failed to descend into the SCROTUM.

undine A glass vessel used for irrigating the eye.

undulant fever see **brucellosis**

ungual Relating to the nails.

unguent An ointment.

unilateral On one side only.

uraemia An excessive amount of urea in the blood, associated with failure of the kidneys.

urea One of the main products resulting from the breakdown of protein in the body. It is excreted by the kidneys into the urine.

ureter The tube passing from the kidney to the bladder. (See URINARY TRACT)

urethra The tube which conveys urine from the urinary bladder to the outside of the body. (See URINARY TRACT)

urethritis Inflammation of the URETHRA.

urinary bladder The collecting sac for the urine which is passed to it by the two ureters from the kidneys. On contraction it expels the urine through the urethra. (See URINARY TRACT)

urinary tract (see page 244)

urinate To pass urine.

urogenital Relating to the urinary and genital systems.

urology The study of the urinary system and the treatment of its diseases.

urticaria An ALLERGIC reaction producing raised red itchy weals on the skin; nettle rash.

uterus The hollow organ situated in the PELVIS in which the fertilized ovum is implanted and develops during pregnancy. (See REPRODUCTIVE SYSTEM, FEMALE)

uveal tract The iris of the eye, the framework supporting it (ciliary body) and the membrane behind the retina (choroid) considered as a whole. (See EYE)

uveitis Inflammation of the uveal tract.

uvula The loose piece of tissue which hangs down from the back of the PALATE.

vaccination 1 INOCULATION with a special VACCINE to protect against SMALLPOX. **2** Inoculation with any vaccine to stimulate the body to produce ANTIBODIES which will make the patient immune or resistant to the infectious disease in question.

V

vaccine A preparation of killed or weakened (attenuated) MICRO-ORGANISMS which, when INOCULATED into the body, will stimulate it to produce ANTIBODIES to protect against the disease caused by those micro-organisms.

urinary tract

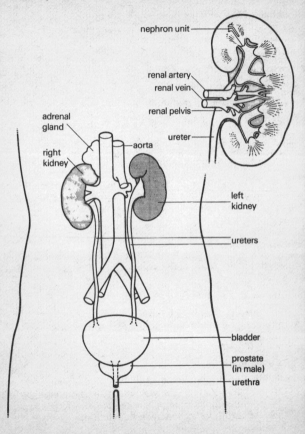

nephron unit

renal artery
renal vein

renal pelvis

ureter

adrenal
gland

aorta

right
kidney

left
kidney

ureters

bladder

prostate
(in male)

urethra

vaccinia Cowpox, a virus infection of cows, similar to but milder than SMALLPOX. A VACCINE from this virus is used to vaccinate against smallpox.

vagal Relating to the VAGUS.

vagina The 'front passage' of the female leading from the VULVA to the opening of the womb. (See REPRODUCTIVE SYSTEM, FEMALE)

vaginismus A painful spasm of the muscles around the vagina, making sexual intercourse impossible or difficult. The cause may be physical or emotional.

vaginitis Inflammation of the VAGINA.

vagotomy Surgical cutting of the VAGUS nerve as a treatment of severe PEPTIC ULCER.

vagus The tenth CRANIAL nerve. Its branches supply the muscles of the LARYNX and throat and regulate the secretions and the muscle tone of organs in the chest and abdomen.

The position of the kidneys, ureters and bladder in the human body. The larger cross-section of the left kidney (top right) shows the blood supply and the position of a nephron unit, extracting from the blood material which will form the urine. This fluid passes into the hollow renal pelvis, which leads to the ureter. From each kidney the ureter passes to and empties into the bladder. Urine is stored here until it has to be passed out through the urethra.

valgus

valgus A deformity in which the part concerned is angled outwards, away from the midline of the body.

valve A membranous flap on the inside of a blood vessel or heart chamber which allows the blood to flow in one direction and prevents backflow.

valvotomy Surgical incision in a VALVE in order to enlarge the aperture where it has become narrowed.

varicella The medical term for CHICKENPOX.

varicocoele Dilation of the veins of the SPERMATIC CORD forming a swelling in the SCROTUM.

varicose veins Lengthened, distended and tortuous veins; a VARIX of veins. They can be found in many parts of the body (see HAEMORRHOIDS, VARICOCOELE) but the term is chiefly used with reference to distended veins at the surface of the legs.

variola see **smallpox**

varix A distended, tortuous blood vessel.

varus A deformity in which the part concerned is angled inwards, towards the midline of the body.

vas (plural, *vasa*) A body tube or vessel.

vascular Relating to the blood vessels.

vascularization The development of new blood vessels in a tissue.

vas deferens The tube through which SPERMATOZOA pass from the epididymis to the urethra. (See REPRODUCTIVE SYSTEM, MALE)

vasectomy Surgical cutting and removal of a section of the VAS DEFERENS as a method of sterilization.

vasoconstriction Narrowing of a blood vessel.

vasodilation Widening of a blood vessel.

vasopressin A HORMONE secreted by the PITUITARY GLAND. It causes VASOCONSTRICTION of small arteries and capillaries and affects the control by the kidneys of the amount of water passed in the urine.

vector An animal, such as an insect, which transmits an infection. Mosquitoes are vectors of malaria.

vein A blood vessel carrying blood from the organs and tissues towards the heart.

vena cava One of the two large veins opening into the right-hand side of the HEART, bringing to it blood from all over the body.

venepuncture The puncturing of a vein with a syringe needle to draw off a blood sample for analysis or to inject a drug into the bloodstream.

venereal disease A disease passed on during sexual activity, for example, SYPHILIS, GONORRHOEA and CHANCROID.

venesection Treatment by incision in a vein to drain off a certain volume of blood.

venom Poison from animals, such as insect stings or snake bites.

venous Relating to the veins.

ventilation The breathing in and out of air at the lungs.

ventral 1 Relating to the abdomen **2** On the abdominal side of the body. (Compare DORSAL)

ventricle A cavity, in particular the ventricles of the brain and the heart. In the heart these are the two major chambers, pumping blood from the right side to the lungs and from the left side to the rest of the body.

ventricular fibrillation A dangerous condition in which the muscles of the ventricles of the HEART cease contracting normally and merely undergo quivering movements. The heart then no longer pumps blood and death is imminent unless immediate help is given. (Compare AURICULAR FIBRILLATION and see also DEFIBRILLATION)

ventriculography A method of taking X-ray pictures of the VENTRICLES of the brain.

venule A very small vein.

vermicide A drug which will kill worms in the intestines.

vermifuge A drug which will expel worms from the intestines.

vernix caseosa A greasy and protective substance found on the skin of a baby at birth.

verruca A wart.

verrucose Having many warts or wartlike excrescences.

version Manipulation of the FOETUS in the womb so as to alter its position and facilitate delivery.

vertebra (plural, *vertebrae*) Any bone of the spine or VERTEBRAL COLUMN. (See SKELETON)

vertebral column The spine or backbone. From its upper end below the skull to its lower tip it is composed of 33 vertebrae. (See SKELETON)

vertex delivery The normal birth of a baby, with the head appearing first.

vertigo Dizziness and loss of balance, with the sensation that the body or its surroundings are moving.

vesical Relating to the bladder.

vesicle A sac-like structure containing fluid.

vesiculation The formation of blisters.

vibrio A genus of curved or comma-shaped bacteria including those of CHOLERA.

villi (singular, *villus*) These are microscopic projections on MUCOUS MEMBRANES, such as are found in the lining of the intestines. They greatly increase the surface area on which digestive processes can take place.

Vincent's angina A bacterial infection of the mouth and throat. It is quite unrelated to ANGINA PECTORIS.

virilism The development in a woman of male secondary sexual characteristics such as facial hair.

virology The study of VIRUSES and the diseases they cause.

virulence The quality of being very poisonous or infectious.

virus The smallest form of micro-organism. In order to live and reproduce it has to be in a living cell.

viscus (plura, *viscera*) Any large organ within the body, excluding those of the nervous, muscular or skeletal systems.

visual acuity Sharpness of vision; the ability to see clearly.

visual field The area of sight covered by one unmoving eye looking straight ahead.

vitamins Organic chemicals present in foods in minute quantities but essential to health. (See pages 251–253)

vitiligo A condition in which patchy areas of skin are without pigment and appear white.

vitreous humour A jelly-like substance within the eyeball. (See EYE)

vocal cords see **larynx**

volar Relating to the sole of the foot or the palm of the hand.

Volkmann's contracture A contraction of the fingers or toes following some deprivation of their blood supply.

volvulus The twisting of a loop of intestine upon itself so that it becomes obstructed.

Von Recklinghausen's disease see **neurofibromatosis**

vulva The external genital organ of the female; the entrance to the VAGINA.

vulvitis Inflammation of the VULVA.

W **wart** A raised hard area on the skin caused by a virus.

Wasserman reaction A blood test for the diagnosis of SYPHILIS. Some other infectious diseases may also produce the same reaction.

wasting The emaciation of an organ or a limb from lack of use, with loss of muscle size.

waters Popular name for AMNIOTIC FLUID.

weal A raised puffy area of skin, with itching, as in cases of URTICARIA.

vitamins

vitamin	good sources	results of deficiency
A (carotene)	dairy products, liver, green leafy vegetables	retarded growth, lowered resistance to infection, dry skin, night blindness, eye disease (xerophthalmia)
B$_1$ (thiamine)	brewer's yeast, whole grain cereals, beans, peas, oranges, liver, kidney, nuts	impaired digestion, colitis, nervous disorders, loss of muscular coordination, beriberi, paralysis
B$_2$ (riboflavine)	eggs, liver, kidney, lean meat, green vegetables, wheat-germ, milk, dried yeast	impaired growth, weakness, inflammation of the tongue, fissured lips, skin disorders, anaemia, cataract, sensitivity to light

vitamins

vitamin	good sources	results of deficiency
niacin (nicotinic acid)	lean meat, fish, yeast, beans, peas, whole grain cereals	pellagra, gastro-intestinal and mental disturbances
B_{12} (cyanocobalamin)	mostly manufactured in man by the action of normal intestinal bacteria; liver, kidney, dairy products	pernicious anaemia
C (ascorbic acid)	fresh fruits and vegetables, citrus juices (especially required for infants, as in orange or tomato juice)	lowered resistance to infection, tender joints, bleeding gums, anaemia, scurvy

vitamins

vitamin	good sources	results of deficiency
D	butter, eggs, liver, fish (salmon, tuna, sardines, herring, oysters), yeast (also formed in the skin when exposed to sunlight)	rickets, osteomalacia
E	green leafy vegetables, margarine, wheatgerm oil, rice	weakening and rupture of the walls of red blood cells
B₆ (pyridoxine)	meat, wheatgerm, cereal grains, black molasses (treacle)	nausea, vomiting, neuritis, skin inflammation around the eyes and mouth
folic acid (folacin)	liver, yeast, green leafy vegetables	anaemia
K	green vegetables, brassicas	bleeding, bruising

Weber test A test used to compare the hearing power of both ears by placing the handle of a vibrating tuning fork in the centre of the forehead.

Weil's disease An infectious illness caused by the bacteria leptospira and transmissible by contact with water or other material contaminated by rats, as in sewers. The illness may be relatively mild, with fever, headache, vomiting and weakness or, in its severe form, may cause kidney troubles, jaundice and a tendency to bleed in different parts of the body.

wen A sebaceous cyst.

whiplash injury An injury to the spine at the neck caused by a sudden jerking backwards and forwards of the head, with stretching, as might happen to a motorist in a collision.

whipworm A type of parasitic roundworm.

white matter see **grey matter**

whitlow Another term for PARONYCHIA.

whooping cough An infection of the respiratory tract, marked by a cough which comes in spasms ending with a sharp, prolonged sound or 'whoop' as breath is drawn in. (See FEVERS OF CHILDHOOD)

Widal reaction A blood test for TYPHOID FEVER and similar infections.

Wilm's tumour Another term for NEPHROBLASTOMA.

Wilson's disease A hereditary disease affecting the liver and some brain centres, causing incoordination of movement and changes in the mental state. It is related to faulty use of copper salts by the body.

wisdom tooth The third molar tooth, which erupts in youth. (See TEETH)

womb see **uterus**

W.R. An abbreviation for WASSERMAN REACTION.

wrist drop Inability to pull the hand up and back at the wrist caused by paralysis of the muscles concerned.

writer's cramp A painful spasm of the muscles of the hand and forearm, associated with the constant repetitive use of the hands for the same task.

wryneck see **torticollis**

xanthelasma XANTHOMA of the eyelids.

xanthoma Nodules in the skin containing soft yellow deposits of fatty substances, including CHOLESTEROL. Found mainly on eyelids and hands, they are often associated with a high amount of cholesterol in the blood.

xanthosis A yellow discoloration of the skin caused by pigments contained in some foods, for example carrots, eaten in large amounts.

X chromosome see **chromosome**

xero- A prefix meaning 'dry'.

xeroderma Abnormal roughness and dryness of the skin.

xerophthalmia Abnormal dryness of the eye.

xiphisternum or **xiphoid process** The free end of bone at the lower end of the sternum. (See SKELETON)

X-rays Electromagnetic waves whose very short wavelengths allows them to pass through the softer TISSUES of the body, although they cannot penetrate harder tissues like bone. Photographs of the results, radiographs, can thus show outlines of structures within the body.

Y **yaws** A chronic contagious disease of tropical regions. It begins with a red pimple, and excrescences and ulcers may subsequently appear anywhere on the skin. If untreated it may in later stages cause damage to bones.

Y chromosome see **chromosome**

yellow atrophy Massive damage to the liver as a result of severe infection or some forms of poisoning.

yellow fever A severe and acute virus infection transmitted by mosquitoes, and found in tropical Africa and South America. It causes damage to the liver, kidneys, stomach and heart, and is accompanied by jaundice.

yersinia pestis BACTERIA which cause PLAGUE.

Z **zo(o)-** A prefix meaning 'relating to animals'.

Zollinger–Ellison syndrome An illness with tumours of the PANCREAS, excess acidity in the stomach and the formation of PEPTIC ULCERS.

zona see **shingles**

zoonoses Diseases of animals which can be transmitted to man.

zygoma The cheekbone. (See SKELETON)

zygote The fertilized OVUM; an ovum fertilized by a SPERMATOZOON.